The Human Ear Canal

Second Edition

The Human Ear Canal

Second Edition

Bopanna B. Ballachanda, PhD

Contributions from:

Richard T. Miyamoto, MD
R. Christopher Miyamoto, MD
Brian Taylor, AuD

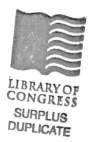
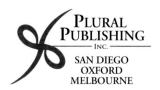

PLURAL
PUBLISHING
INC.

SAN DIEGO
OXFORD
MELBOURNE

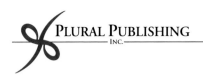

5521 Ruffin Road
San Diego, CA 92123

e-mail: info@pluralpublishing.com
Web site: http://www.pluralpublishing.com

Typeset in 11/13 Palatino by Flanagan's Publishing Services, Inc.
Printed in the United States of America by Bang Printing

Library of Congress Cataloging-in-Publication Data

Ballachanda, Bopanna B.
  The human ear canal / Bopanna B. Ballachanda ; contributions from Richard
T. Miyamoto, Christopher Miyamoto, Brian Taylor. — 2nd ed.
       p. ; cm.
  Includes bibliographical references and index.
  ISBN-13: 978-1-59756-413-7 (alk. paper)
  ISBN-10: 1-59756-413-3 (alk. paper)
  I. Miyamoto, Richard T. II. Miyamoto, Christopher. III. Taylor, Brian, 1966-
IV. Title.
  [DNLM: 1. Ear Canal. WV 222]
  LC Classification not assigned
  617.8'3 — dc23
                    2012043307

Contents

Preface

At first one might wonder about the need for a second edition of the textbook on *The Human Ear Canal*. The answer is straightforward; after the publication of the first edition, a large body of research articles have been published in many scientific journals to enrich our understanding of the ear canal, its secretory functions, cerumen management, and acoustics. Thus, the second edition of the book provides the current knowledge that will be beneficial to specialists in many disciplines. The ear canal, a skin-lined tube, is an important structure of our auditory system that has been studied by otologists, audiologists, physicists, geneticists, and others. The ear canal needs to be understood so that manipulative procedures can be carried out efficiently in the ear canal itself, and the canal is also an important path to gain access to the middle ear.

This second edition of the *The Human Ear Canal* arose from the need to inform audiologists about the current understanding of the human ear canal and its importance to audiological services. The goals of the first edition was to: (1) discuss the anatomy and physiology of the ear canal and the importance of ear canal measurements in audiological diagnosis, (2) examine the relationship between the ear canal and hearing aid fittings, and (3) provide a guide to cerumen management. The goal of the second edition is not only to update the first edition but also to incorporate evidence and value-based perspectives while performing cerumen management.

As mentioned in the first edition, audiologists are constantly probing the ear canal for placement of earphones, microphones, electrodes, and other devices during the evaluation of the auditory and vestibular systems. Several measurements performed within the canal include probe microphone insertion for real-ear measurements during hearing aid selection and fitting, otoacoustic emission testing, and immittance measurements. In addition, inserted earphones are used routinely to deliver sounds during hearing testing. Despite a great interest in conducting measurements within the ear canal, little attention has been focused on the importance of the status of the ear canal, which can alter the stimulus being delivered; this books addresses the significance of the ear canal during these measurements.

Even though I have a broad understanding of the ear canal, I felt the need to seek contributions from several renowned specialists in related fields to provide a detailed account of the ear canal. Chapters by Dr. Richard T. Miyamoto and Dr. R. Christopher Miyamoto, noted otologists, help us understand the anatomy and pathology of the ear canal. To create an independent and caring profession audiologists must recognize pathologies of the ear canal in order to serve their patients effectively by referring them to appropriate medical facilities for prompt medical attention when needed. Dr. Taylor is not a newcomer to the field of audiology and hearing aids; his contributions to the field of audiology are considerable. He has published books, chapters, and articles on hearing aids. The chapter by Dr. Taylor gives us a better understanding of the relationship between the ear canal and hearing aids.

It is in the spirit of cooperative endeavor that the present work is offered, so that the audiologists can appreciate the contributions to the understanding of the ear canal from several disciplines. The second edition has been under development for about two years, and every attempt has been made to incorporate recent developments in this book. Writing a book is not an easy task, but the time spent in preparing it will be richly rewarded when audiologists begin to further their appreciation of the complexity of the human ear canal and make use of this information in their research and clinical practice.

Acknowledgments

I owe a debt of gratitude to Dr. Sadanand Singh for encouraging me to write this second edition. Even though Dr. Singh is not present, the same level of support and enthusiasm has been provided by Mrs. Angie Singh and I am very indebted to her. I also want to thank several past and current employees at Plural Publishing for their unwavering support. The one person who wanted to see this book published and who is no longer with us is Sandy Doyle—she deserves a special thank you for her work on the first edition and the early part of the second edition. Several members of the Plural team deserve my heartfelt appreciation; they are Caitlin Mahon for painstakingly reading the manuscript and meticulously editing the chapters, and Valerie Johns for her leadership to get the book published on a timely basis.

I have a special debt of gratitude to Mr. Robert Everett, an engineer by training but who was involved in measuring vocal tract acoustics and had a great understanding of acoustics in curved tubes; he helped me with various equations used in Chapter 6. Special thanks are to Dr. Muller, clinical associate professor at the University of Arizona, for taking time to review Chapter 9; and Mike Ryan, president of Preferred Product, for helping with several cerumen management workshops and also supplying with several illustrations in this book. A very special thanks to Vanessa Sawyer, my executive assistant, for helping me with keeping track of the progress of the book from the beginning to its completion.

I wish to extend my heartfelt appreciation to my family for allowing me to spend a large segment of evenings writing this book: to my wife Naina Ballachanda, son Tanek Ballachanda, and daughter Jyothi Ballachanda for their understanding, patience, and support. Last but not least I owe a special thanks to all the international, national, state, and other organizations for inviting me to present lecturers on the ear canal and cerumen management, which has helped me considerably in organizing this book.

Contributors

Bopanna B. Ballachanda, PhD
CEO—Board Certified Audiologist
Premier Hearing Centers
Arizona, New Mexico, and Texas
Chapters 1, 2, 4, 6, 8, and 9

Richard T. Miyamoto, MD, FACS, FAAP
Arilla Spence DeVault Professor and Chairman
Department of Otolaryngology-Head and Neck Surgery
Indiana University School of Medicine
Indianapolis, Indiana
Chapters 3 and 5

R. Christopher Miyamoto, MD, FACS, FAAP
Pediatric Otolaryngology
Peyton Manning Children's Hospital at St. Vincent
Indianapolis, Indiana
Chapters 3 and 5

Brian Taylor, AuD
Director, Practice Development and Clinical Affairs
Unitron Hearing Systems
Chapter 7

In memory of:
Ballachanda C. Belliappa
and
George Moushegian, PhD

1

Introduction

BOPANNA B. BALLACHANDA

The Human Ear Canal

The human ear canal is a skin-lined cul-de-sac that extends from the concha of the auricle to the tympanic membrane. The ear canal and the outer ear are special parts of the hearing mechanism seen only in certain mammals. Its primary function is to serve as a conduit for the passage of sound waves to the tympanic membrane. It also functions to protect the middle and inner ear from external trauma by impeding the entry of foreign objects and by correcting fluctuations in environmental temperatures.

Study of the Human Ear Canal

The human ear canal has been a topic of considerable interest across several disciplines. Dermatologists have studied this tube with great curiosity as it is the only skin-lined cavity in the body. Because it is a skin-lined cavity, the treatment of ear canal diseases has followed the principles of the treatment of dermotoses of the rest of the body. Otologists have a special interest in the ear canal because it serves as the only avenue through which to evaluate the status of the middle and inner ear, and it is an access point during surgery of the middle ear. Anthropologists have investigated the secretory product known as cerumen in attempts to unearth genetic traits among different racial groups. Hearing scientists are intrigued by the ear canal pressure gain (also known as the resonant frequency) at various frequencies compared to free-field sound.

The ear canal continues to play an important role in audiological diagnosis and treatment. This book has combined all the scientific advances in ear canal measurements to provide a cohesive account of the ear canal, particularly as it relates to audiology. Audiologists have incorporated ear canal measurements as part of the audiologic diagnosis while evaluating the hearing status of patients, the transfer function of the middle ear, and functions of the inner ear through otoacoustic emission, electrocochleaography, and auditory brainstem responses. In addition, ear canals have served as anchors for hearing aids of all shapes and sizes. Thus, the ear canal is an important part of audiology.

Human Ear Canal in Thermometry

Even though William and Thomson (1948) reported that the ear canal was a possible site for the measurement of body temperature in humans, it was not until the 1960s that the ear canal was studied as a potential site for monitoring the body temperature of spacecraft crew during preflight and in flight testing. The need for a reliable site for monitoring body temperature variations in manned flights over a long period of time other than through oral and rectal locations became obvious. The oral and rectal temperature measuring-devices were either uncomfortable or objectionable over long periods of measurements. The ear canal was chosen as an accessible and suitable site for measuring core body temperature because the tympanic membrane is supplied with blood from the carotid artery, which also supplies blood to the hypothalamus, the temperature regulatory system in the human body. Furthermore, the ear canal has a temperature gradient with its highest temperature closest to the tympanic membrane and its lowest at the entrance of the ear canal, as illustrated in Figure 1–1. Gibbons (1967) compared ear canal temperature to that of oral and reported that the ear canal was a suitable place to monitor body temperature.

Advances in design and improvement in accuracy of thermometry helped establish the ear canal as a reliable site to measure body temperature. Developments in the technology of thermometry allow the assessment of body temperature by measuring the infrared emission from the ear canal and tympanic membrane. Among the sites identified for temperature measurements, the ear canal and tympanic membrane have

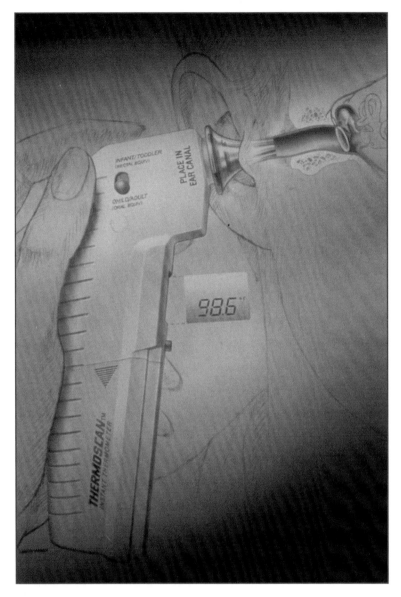

Figure 1–1. *Illustration of temperature variations inside the ear canal. (Courtesy of Thermoscan®, Inc.)*

gained rapid acceptance among pediatricians, physicians, and nurses. Ear canal and tympanic membrane thermometry offers the advantages of ease of monitoring, speed of use, improved hygiene, greater patient satisfaction, and convenience.

This type of ear thermometer is called an infrared emission detection (IRED) thermometer, one of the commercially available IRED, also known as infrared tympanic thermometer (IRTT), is shown in Figure 1–2. When

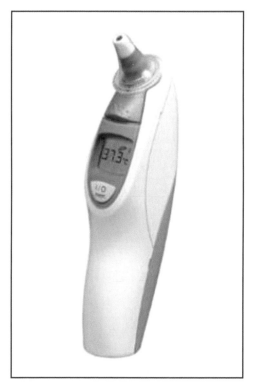

Figure 1–2. *Image of an infrared ear thermometer. (Courtesy of Radiant®)*

the IRT thermometer is properly oriented inside the canal and activated, the probe collects the naturally occurring electromagnetic radiation emission from the tympanic membrane and the surrounding area.

The instrument may measure emission as a "snap shot" in which shutters open briefly, or as a "scan" in which the probe scans the temperature for about five seconds. After taking the measurement, the thermometer displays the temperature using several algorithms developed by each manufacturer. The IRTT is a newer concept compared to rectal and oral cavity locations to gather body temperature. Despite the fact that it is easy to use, recent studies have questioned the accuracy of the temperature measurements obtained by IRTT devices. Following the introduction of commercially available IRTT devices, Yaron et al. (1995) compared the IRTT temperature measurement to that of rectal temperature readings to determine the accuracy of the new device (IRTT) to that of traditional measurement (rectal); and also to determine the accuracy of detecting fever in their patient population. They concluded that the differences existed between the two devices and the accuracy to detect fever was only 60%, therefore, it was unsatisfactory to completely rely on

IRTT. They also noted that cerumen impaction and the presence of otitis media can lead to errors in measurement. Daanen (2006) stated that the morphology, specifically the circumference of the ear canal is another factor that can confound the accuracy temperature measurements along with cerumen impaction and middle ear pathologies. A recent study by Twerenbold et al. (2010) examined 333 patients to determine the effect of cerumen impaction on body temperature measurements. Although cerumen impaction caused a statistically significant difference, it did not have a clinically meaningful influence on intra ear temperature measurement (IETM). Thus, routine ear inspection prior to the use of IETM is not warranted. They concluded that IETM provides highly reproducible assessments of infrared ear temperature (IET) irrespective of penetration depth, side of measurement, and acclimatization.

Although thermometry has not been an area of concern to most audiologists in the past, the fact that this instrument is being placed in the ear canal should raise questions relating to cerumen impaction, health, hygiene, and potential trauma to the ear canal that are inherent with hearing aids, earmolds, and many of the test procedures currently employed by audiologists. Thus, at least territorially, this topic may hold more interest for audiologists in the future. It certainly is an example of how interest and interaction with the ear canal continues to evolve from both inside and outside of our field and helps establish the need for audiologists to know as much as possible about the ear canal and its function in order to stay current with this aspect of their profession. Therefore, it also helps establish, and is a further example of, why this book should be a prerequisite for all audiologists, physicians, and others interested in the ear.

Cerumen Management

A driving force to write the second edition of this book was the need to update many chapters in light of new data being added and a renewed interest in cerumen management (Roland et al., 2008) by audiologists and other health care professionals. When the first edition was published, cerumen management was an emerging concept for audiologists, many were concerned that cerumen management required considerable training and education; worried about the possibility of adverse effects, even though several audiologists and hearing health care providers were already engaged in cerumen management in their practices, many were hesitant to incorporate the procedure into their clinical practice. The first edition provided a conformation to all the clinicians that cerumen management is part of the audiology practice and those who were hesitant acquired a well-designed program through workshops at national and state level meeting to incorporate cerumen management into their clinical armamentarium. At present, the concerns and hesitancy that prevailed during the early phase of cerumen management has lessened partly because it is now being taught in doctoral programs as part of their course work and clinical practicum. In addition, a number of articles have provided scientific evidence that performing cerumen management is safe and effective with good clinical judgment and proper training. Another major change seen in audiology practice is our ability to make clinical decisions on cerumen management based on evidence and value-based information.

Evidence-Based Practice

Audiologists and audiology clinics have recognized the need to implement evidence and value-based practices. At present health care providers strongly believe that learning evidence-based practices improves the efficacy with which health care providers gather and process new and meaningful information during their career. Once the clinician learns the importance of evidence-based practice, the practitioner will be able to differentiate the levels of evidence for intervention to facilitate delivery of the highest quality of care. In addition to appreciating the scientific merit of the procedures that the clinician follows, they are also able to distill the article's information based on merits and not simply or blindly accept an article at face value. A summary of the levels of evidence described in several books and journals is in Table 1–1. A detailed description of meta-analysis and evidence-based information on cerumen management is explained in Chapter 9.

Value-Based Practice

In evidence-based practice the outcome is determined by the quality of evidence and the balance of benefit and harm. The value-based statement or outcome is determined by the improvement of the quality of life following a procedure. At present, there are very limited value based instruments in audiology to assess the improvement in quality of life by the intervention of a therapeutic procedure. Stated differently, the value-based practice is focused on the patient-perceived value conferred by an

Table 1–1. Level of Evidence for Review of Studies in This Book Ranked According to Quality of Evidence from Highest to Lowest

Level/Grade	Quality of Evidence—Description of Evidence
I	Well-designed study that uses randomized controls and incorporates meta analysis. Low type-1 error (≤ 0.05) and low type-2 error (≤ 0.20).
II	Well-designed, randomized control study with minor limitations—Overwhelmingly consistent evidence. High type-1 error (>0.05) and/or high type-2 error (>0.20).
III	Well-designed but uncontrolled, nonrandomized study. Observational studies (treatment group compared to no treatment group in a nonrandomized study).
IV	Well-designed but quasi-experimental study that includes: expert opinion, case reports, reasoning from animal studies. Also can be intervention on several patients without a comparison group.
V	Exceptional situations where well-designed studies cannot be performed, single case report, nonexperimental studies, study explains benefit from harm.
X	Committee reports, conference reports, clinical experiences from noted person in the field.

intervention. The best value-based practice should take the evidence-based data and apply it towards value form. The value-based practice should also confer the resources expanded on a given intervention and its outcome. In the field of audiology, value based practice should review the time spent on evidence-based protocol to arrive at an intervention and its perceived value by the patient. It would be ideal to have an instrument/scale that can convert the evidence-based data to patient-perceived value using a common outcome measure. The common practice to convert the evidence-based data to value-based data is by using utility analysis, and the cost-utility analysis will provide the cost associated with the intervention.

In spite of important developments in implementing cerumen management within the practice of audiology, there are no specific requirements or guidelines available at the present time. The chapter on cerumen management strives to provide an evidence-based guideline for all clinicians; however, it is left to the clinician to determine the value based outcome from their patient perceived benefits. Proficiency in cerumen management requires good clinical judgment and appropriate training. A well-trained and experienced clinician will minimize traumatic and inadequate extraction. Unless audiologists accept responsibility for cerumen management, they will seriously limit their services to a large percentage of their patient population. For audiologists to be independent practitioners, they must accept the responsibility of cerumen management. Cerumen management associated with other procedures will increase the accessibility of audiologic practices to the public and increase the use of their audiologic services.

Organization of the Text

The chapters in this book cover a wide range of topics pertinent to the human ear canal and its contribution to audiological services. The embryonic development of the ear canal and further alterations due to progressive changes in aging are discussed in the second chapter. The third chapter describes the shape, size, neural innervations, and vascular supply to the ear canal. The illustrations in this chapter provide an enhanced view of the various structures within the ear canal. The fourth chapter emphasizes the need for good visualization of the ear canal during examination. The ability to identify various medical and non-medical conditions is important for audiologists in order to qualify themselves as independent practitioners and to practice audiology with greater confidence. A comprehensive visualization of the ear canal is important for both diagnosis and treatment.

The fifth chapter deals with pathological conditions of the ear canal. Audiologists are well-trained professionals and can serve as a point of entry to the hearing health care system. Sullivan (1993) stated that, "what the eyeball is functionally to the optometrist, the external ear is functionally similar to the audiologist." It is not the intent of this book to advocate that audiologists should diagnose medical conditions, but they should identify medical conditions for referral to physicians for better patient management.

Chapter 6 describes various techniques to determine ear canal geometry, the importance of sound pressure measurements within the ear canal, and the variables affecting ear canal measurements. An attempt is made to gather all the relevant publications in the area of ear canal measurements so that students and audiologists need not spend countless hours searching numerous journals to keep up with the rapid development in measurements performed within the ear canal. Chapter 7 emphasizes the relationship between the hearing aid and the ear canal; the importance of the ear canal and its associated structures for successful hearing aid fitting are also discussed.

Chapters 8 and 9 are devoted to the physiology/pathophysiology of cerumen and procedures for cerumen management. Excessive cerumen can be a problem for hearing professionals and their patients. Its presence can interfere with patient testing and make it impossible to obtain reliable test results or obtain a precise ear canal impression. The normal course of cerumen production, the causes and prevalence of cerumen impaction, the consequences of cerumen accumulation on audiological diagnosis, and the precise procedures for cerumen management are detailed in these chapters.

2

Developmental Anatomy of the Outer Ear

BOPANNA B. BALLACHANDA

INTRODUCTION

The developmental aspects of the human ear canal reflect changes that span from the embryonic period of fetal development to those that occur in older ears later in life. Remarkable and continual changes in size, shape, and dimension of the ear take place during the prenatal stage compared to those that occur in childhood and adulthood. Consequently, the emphasis of this chapter is predominantly on the mechanism of embryogenesis that is responsible for the formation of the ear canal and pinna from conception to childhood. The information covered in this chapter is drawn from several books and articles (Altman, 1950; Anson, 1980; Gulya, 1990; Kenna, 1990; Nishimura & Kumoi, 1992; Sperber, 1994; Streeter, 1922; Van De Water, Noden, & Maderson, 1988; Williams, 1994). Most of the information presented in this chapter is dated because of the fact that study of human development was of great interest in the early part of the 20th century. However, the information is still valid and accurate, and therefore very few investigators have revisited this topic in recent years to reconfirm the previous findings and add new data from improved technical knowledge.

The impetus to study the embryogenesis of the ear stems from a need to better understand the relationship between forms of dysmorphology that are exhibited in many congenital anomalies occurring at different developmental stages. For example, an insult during the early gestational period may result in damage to the pinna and ear canal, but may not affect the middle ear structures or the inner ear. Others can affect all parts of the ear, and noticeable deviations of the outer ear may reflect abnormalities of the other structures as well.

This chapter is dedicated to the understanding of anatomical changes of the outer ear; however, other considerations such as subcellular biochemical mechanisms, histogenesis, and morphogenesis should be borne in mind for a detailed understanding of this enormous field of study known as "Embryology." Interestingly, Northern and Downs (1992) stated that "most audiologists have not had training or course work in the field of embryology, so some basic background information is essential to appreciate fully the development of the ear" (p. 35).

A first step toward understanding the development of the ear canal is to provide a basic coverage of the early part of the embryonic development (i.e., from conception to initial differentiation of ear canal and pinna/auricle). Succeeding conception (i.e., the spermatozoon penetrating the ovum to form the zygote), the cells divide through a process known as mitosis, whereby identical cells are formed from pre-existing cells. At the same time, due to differentiation processes, the embryo forms three layers known as the ectoderm, mesoderm, and endoderm. These three layers are the bases of all organ and structural formations. The various structural derivatives from these three layers are shown in Figure 2–1 and listed in Table 2–1. It is apparent that the ectoderm layer is responsible for the development of the outer and inner ear whereas the ossicles and bone surrounding the inner ear originate from the mesoderm layer.

Development of the Auricle/Pinna

During the fourth week of gestation, the auricle develops from the first and second branchial arches, also known as the mandibular and hyoid arches. These arches are located at the dorsal extremity of the first branchial grove as tissue growths or thickenings, as shown in Figure 2–2. At about the same time, the development of the inner ear takes place through the formation of auditory vesicles located dorsal to the hyoid vesicles and second branchial groove. Chronologically, during the fifth

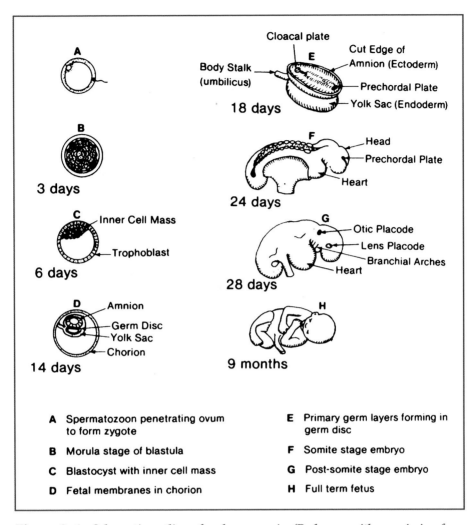

Figure 2–1. *Schematic outline of embryogenesis. (Redrawn with permission from G. H. Sperber. Embryology of the head and neck. In G. M. English [Ed.], 1988. Oto-laryngology, Vol. I, Diseases of the Ear and Hearing. Rev. ed. Philadelphia, PA: J. B. Lippincott Company).*

and sixth week, tissue thickens or condenses on both sides of the first branchial groove to form the six hillocks, arising equally from the mandibular and hyoid arches as described by His (1885) and illustrated in Figure 2–3, at 14 mm in length (5+ weeks), these hillocks lie close to each other, and as the auricle develops (end of sixth week), they are pushed apart and fuse around the branchial groove to form two folds. The anterior fold is derived from the mandibular arch and the posterior fold from the hyoid arch. Furthermore, these six hillocks are believed to be responsible for the growth of the external ear including the shape and

Table 2–1. Primary Germ Layers: Ectoderm, Mesoderm, and Endoderm and the Various Parts Derived From These Layers

Ectoderm		Mesoderm	Endoderm
Neural Crest	**Neural Tissue**	**Mesoderm**	**Endoderm**
Leptomeninges	Brain and nerves	Connective tissues (bone, cartilage, blood)	Auditory tube and tympanum lining
Nerve ganglia	Cutaneous derivatives		
Neural sheath cells	Skin (epidermis: sweat glands, mammary glands, sebaceous glands, hair, nails)	Muscle	Epithelia of the pharynx trachea, bronchi, lungs
Adrenal medulla		Dermis	
Melanocytes		Urogenital system	
Autonomic nerves		Spleen	Gut lining
Scleral and choroid optic coats	Dental enamal	Adrenal cortex	Visceral parenchyma (liver, pancreas)
Branchial arches			Urinary bladder
Lining			Tonsils
Skull bones			Parathyroids
Dental pulp			Thymus
Dentin			
Periodontal ligament			
Portions of thymus			
Calcitonin "C" cells			
Carotid body			
Portions of heart			

Source: Reproduced with permission from: G. H. Sperber. Embryology of the head and neck. In G. M. English (Ed.), *Otolaryngology*. Philadelphia, PA: J. B. Lippincott Company.

size. Streeter (1922) was quite concerned that considerable emphasis had been placed on these hillocks; he believed that the hillocks are transitory and incidental in nature rather than fundamental to the formation of the auricle.

The exact adult structures that form from these hillocks are controversial; however, the more widely accepted view is that the auricle is

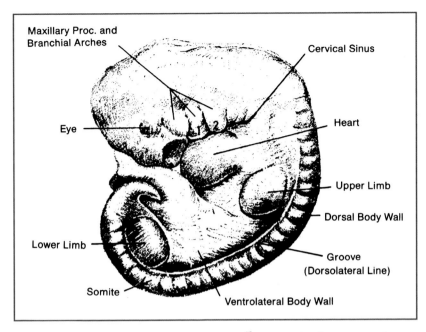

Figure 2–2. *Lateral view of the embryo showing the formation of mandibular and hyoid arches also known as branchial arches 1 and 2. (Redrawn with permission from G. H. William. Developmental anatomy of the ear. In G. M. English [Ed.], 1988.* Otolaryngology, Vol. I, Diseases of the Ear and Hearing. *Rev. ed. Philadelphia, PA: J. B. Lippincott Company).*

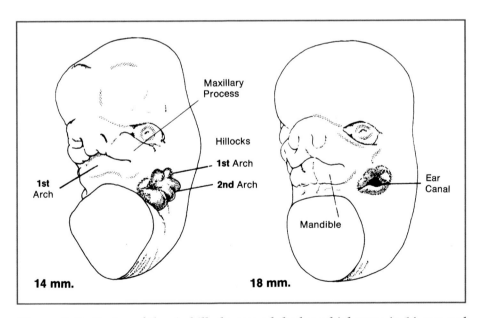

Figure 2–3. *Fusion of the six hillocks around the branchial grove in 14-mm and 18-mm embryo. (Redrawn with permission from G. H. William. Developmental anatomy of the ear. In G. M. English [Ed.], 1988.* Otolaryngology, Vol. I, Diseases of the Ear and Hearing. *Rev. ed. Philadelphia, PA: J. B. Lippincott Company).*

developed from the second branchial arch (hyoid arch) whereas the tragus originates from the first branchial arch (mandibular arch). Schematics of the contributions of the hyoid and mandibular arches are shown in Figure 2–4. The auricle, derived from the first (mandibular) arch, is larger in the younger stages, than the parts developed from the second (hyoid) arch; however, as the fetus grows (i.e., when it is 85 mm long at 3 months of gestation), the parts originating from the second (hyoid) arch are greater compared to the previous stages (Wood-Jones & Wen, 1934). The formation of the auricle from the six hillocks is illustrated in Figure 2–5 and summarized as follows: the first hillock gives rise to the region of the tragus, the second hillock forms the crus of the helix, the third hillock develops into the majority of the helix, the fourth hillock becomes the antihelix; the fifth hillock leads to the antitragus, and finally the sixth hillock forms the lobule and lower part of the helix. As a result of the different origin of these hillocks, innervations vary between them. The first three from the mandibular arch are innervated by the mandibular division of the fifth cranial nerve, and the remaining three are innervated by several nerve fibers including the facial nerve and branches of cervical plexus. The concha is formed from the middle and upper parts of the branchial groove. From the seventh week to the twentieth week the auricle continues to develop; at the twentieth week the auricle assumes the adult configuration; during the same time frame, the auricle position starts shifting from the ventromedial to the dorsolateral location, as a result of mandibular and facial growth. The tubercle, also known as Darwin's tubercle, is evident in the sixth month; there are considerable normal variations in the size and shape of Darwin's tubercle and these differences have been attributed to the developmental variations in the six hillocks. Cartilage is formed by the seventh week from the folds of mesenchyme. The newborn auricle is smaller compared to the adult, and the cartilage of the pinna is soft and pliable. The auricle attains adult shape by the age of nine years, and by that time cartilage becomes firmer and histologically mature.

Additionally, the mesoderm in the hyoid arch helps to develop the auricular muscles to attach the pinna to the scalp and head. These muscles are responsible for the movement of the auricle as a whole in animals for directional hearing. In humans, these muscles are functionally insignificant. A survey of congenital anomalies of the auricle suggests that the most commonly observed problem is the absence or incomplete formation of pinna known as microtia-anotia; these anomalies have been attributed to incomplete fusion of the hillocks, mostly between the tragus and antitragus. A detailed discussion of pathology of the outer ear is presented in Chapter 5.

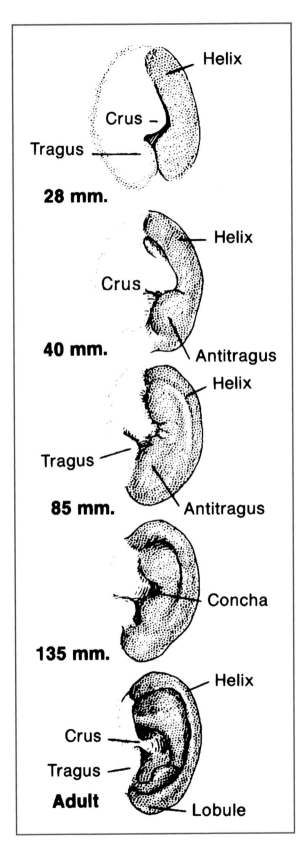

Figure 2–4. *Diagrammatic representation of the parts of the auricle developed from the mandibular arch* (lighter area) *and the parts derived from the hyoid arch* (darker area). *The area developed from the mandibular arch is larger in younger stages compared to the parts developed from hyoid arches. The approximate ages are, 8 weeks (28 mm), 9 weeks (40 mm), 3 months (85 mm), 4 months (135 mm), and adult auricle. (Redrawn with permission from G. H. William. Developmental anatomy of the ear. In G. M. English [Ed.], 1988.* Otolaryngology, Vol. I, Diseases of the Ear and Hearing. *Rev. ed. Philadelphia, PA: J. B. Lippincott Company).*

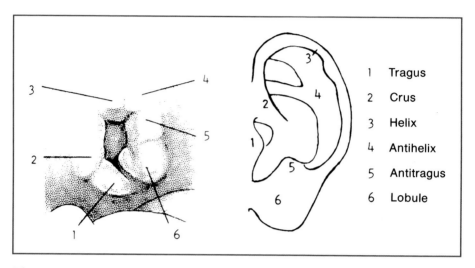

Figure 2–5. *Diagrammatic interpretation of auricular development from the six hillocks. Six hillocks in a 13-mm embryo (6 weeks' gestation). Formation of the auricle from six hillocks. (Redrawn with permission from G. H. William. Developmental anatomy of the ear. In G. M. English [Ed.], 1988. Otolaryngology, Vol. I, Diseases of the Ear and Hearing. Rev. ed. Philadelphia, PA: J.B. Lippincott Company).*

Development of the Ear Canal

The ear canal is derived from the dorsal part of the first branchial groove, which is located between the mandibular and hyoid arches during the fourth to fifth week of gestation. In the second month of gestation, the dorsal part deepens to form a funnel-shaped depression. From the fourth to fifth week, the ectoderm of the first branchial groove is in brief contact with the endodermal lining of the pharyngeal pouch as illustrated in Figure 2–6A. Then the mesodermal tissue subsequently grows between the pharyngeal pouch (tubotympanum) and the branchial groove and separates these two layers (Figure 2–6B). The branchial groove deepens further toward the middle ear during the eighth week to form the primary/primitive meatus which is shown is Figure 2–6C. The funnel shaped indentation in Figure 2–6C becomes the outer cartilaginous part of the ear canal. At this time the entire ear canal is made of cartilaginous segments only.

The ectodermal groove continues to grow from the outside toward the middle ear until it meets with the epithelium of the pharyngeal pouch as shown in Figure 2–7: a cord of thickened epithelial cells, which has arisen from the surface ectoderm, called the meatal plate, extends from the canal to the lower part of the tympanic cavity, and finally the

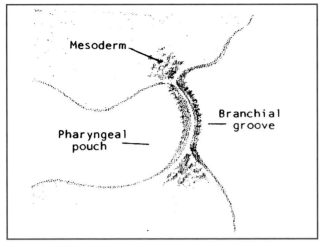

A

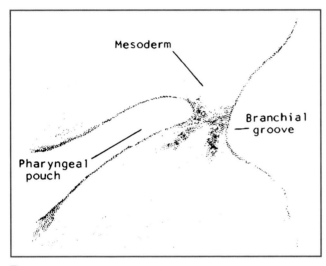

B

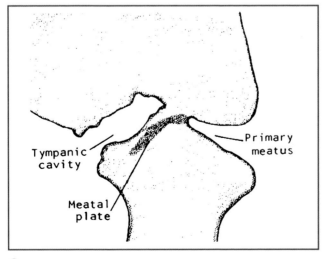

C

Figure 2–6. Draw-
ings illustrating the
relationship between
the branchail groove
and the pharyngeal
pouch. **A.** At the 5th
week, the brachial
groove invaginates
medially toward the
pharyngeal pouch.
B. The mesoderm
grows between the
branchail groove and
the pharyngeal pouch
(6-week embryo).
C. At eight weeks,
formation of primary/
primitive ear canal
and the tympanic
cavity. (Redrawn with
permission from G. H.
William. Developmen-
tal anatomy of the ear.
In G. M. English [Ed.],
1988. Otolaryngology,
Vol. I, Diseases of
the Ear and Hearing.
*Rev. ed. Philadelphia,
PA: J. B. Lippincott
Company*).

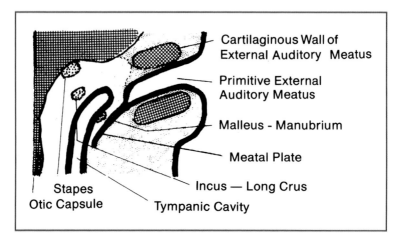

Figure 2–7. *Development of primary ear canal and meatal plate in relation to tympanic cavity at 9 weeks' gestation. (Redrawn with permission from G. H. William. Developmental anatomy of the ear. In G. M. English [Ed.], 1988.* Otolaryngology, Vol. I, Diseases of the Ear and Hearing. *Rev. ed. Philadelphia, PA: J. B. Lippincott Company).*

meatal plate terminates as a round disklike swelling. Mesanchyme grows between the meatal plate and the epithelial layer to form the fibrous layer of the tympanic membrane. The three layers of the tympanic membrane consisting of the inner circular fibers, the fibrous middle layers, and the outer radial fibers are developed by the ninth week of gestation. The meatal plug discussed earlier, and shown in Figure 2–8, remains closed until the 21st week (Williams, 1988). The central part of the meatal plug disintegrates to form a canal. The innermost segment forms the superficial layer of the tympanic membrane as seen in Figure 2–8.

The nontympanic part is the precursor of the bony section of the adult auditory canal. By the seventh month, the inner two-thirds of the ear canal is formed. Controversy exists regarding the actual time frame of canal development; some have pointed out that it is complete by the 21st week, and others believe the time to be at 28 weeks. To resolve the differences in the time course of development, Nishimura and Kumoi (1992) examined several human specimens from eight weeks to 21 weeks. Surprisingly, their findings suggested that the ear canal is morphologically completed by the 18th week, and the tympanic membrane is completely developed by the 21st week. One hopes that additional studies will shed further light into the actual time and support the findings of Nishimura and Kumoi (1992).

The development of the auricle cartilage helps form the walls of the outer two-thirds of the ear canal. At the same time, it is believed

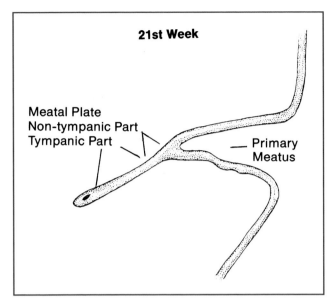

Figure 2–8. *Illustration of meatal plate and the precursor (nontympanic part) of the inner two-thirds section. (Redrawn with permission from G. H. William. Developmental anatomy of the ear. In G. M. English [Ed.], 1988.* Otolaryngology, Vol. I, Diseases of the Ear and Hearing. *Rev. ed. Philadelphia, PA: J. B. Lippincott Company).*

that ceruminous glands and hair follicles develop on the epithelial lining along the cartilaginous part of the canal. The lining of the ear canal and the outer epithelium of the tympanic membrane are ectodermal in origin (Van der Water, Maderson, & Jaskoll, 1980). There is little information in the literature regarding the fetal development of cerumen glands. The only definitive study done 60 years ago by Simonetta and Magnoni (1937) described the appearance of sebaceous glands by the 17th week along with the development of hair follicles. According to these findings, modified apocrine glands are recognized shortly thereafter. Wright (1997) identified the presence of both apocrine and sebaceous glands by the age of 22 gestational weeks in humans (Figure 2–9) and a more mature configuration is shown in Figure 2–10 at 28 weeks in the gestational period (Wright, 1997). Both types of glands appear structurally complete by the age of 6 months gestational age.

The newborn ear canal measures around 20 mm in length; it is shallow, straight, and the entire canal is cartilaginous. Perry mentions in his book that in young children, hair follicles may be present up to the tympanic membrane as the ear canal is still cartilaginous (*The Human Ear Canal*, 1957; p. 7). A comparative view of the newborn and adult ear canal

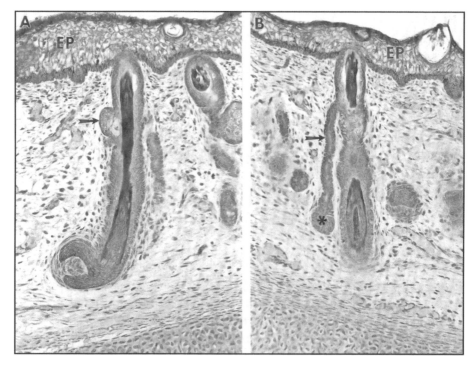

Figure 2–9. *Hair follicles with associated glands in the lateral portion of the external auditory canal of a 22-week gestational age human fetus.* **A.** *A developing sebaceous gland (arrow) budding from the upper portion of a hair follicle.* **B.** *A differentiating modified apocrine gland (asterisk) with its secretory duct (arrow) entering a hair follicle. EP = epidermis on the surface of the ear canal. (Reproduced with permission from C. G. Wright, 1997. Development of the human external ear.* Journal of the American Academy of Audiology, 8[6], 379–390).

and tympanic membrane is shown in Figure 2–11. In addition, in the newborn, the tympanic ring is not completely closed; the ends are connected at that time by the lower border of the temporal squama. Much of the definitive form of the ear canal is complete by the first year of birth; however, adult size is not reached until seven years of age. During the first three years, bony formation takes place in the unossified fibrous plate of the inner two-thirds of the ear canal to become the osseous part. It is at this time that the tympanic membrane orientation changes to look more like that of adults and the canal assumes the adult S-shape. The angle of the tympanic membrane approximates 50 to 60 degrees compared to the infant tympanic membrane, which is oblique or horizontal.

The most critical period for the development of the outer ear is during the first three months of pregnancy; any insult or disease may result

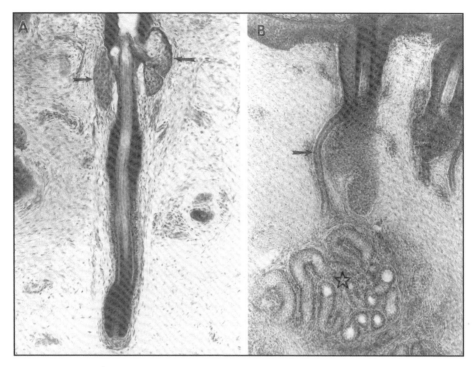

Figure 2–10. *Later stages of external auditory canal gland development.* **A.** *Sebaceous glands (arrows) attached to a hair follicle in a 28-week gestational age human fetus. Coiled tubules of a modified apocrine gland (star) in a 1-year-old infant. The secretory duct (arrow) of the gland is seen opening into a hair follicle. (Reproduced with permission from C. G. Wright, 1997. Development of the human external ear.* Journal of the American Academy of Audiology, 8[6], 379–390).

in alterations in the formation of the ear canal and pinna. Atresia of the ear canal may result from a failure in the formation of a meatal epithelial plug or from a lack of canalization of the meatal plug. Meatal atresia may be either membranous or osseous. The atresia of the inner two-thirds osseous region is more common and it is usually accompanied by middle ear malformations.

Table 2–2 recapitulates development of the outer ear over time. The first branchial arch (mandibular) gives rise to the tragus and the crus of the helix. The remaining structures of the auricle are formed from the second branchial arch (hyoid). A portion of the first branchial groove develops into the ear canal. Although the ear canal and pinna assumes adult form at the time of birth, these two structures continue to grow until seven to nine years of age, at which time adult shape and size is attained.

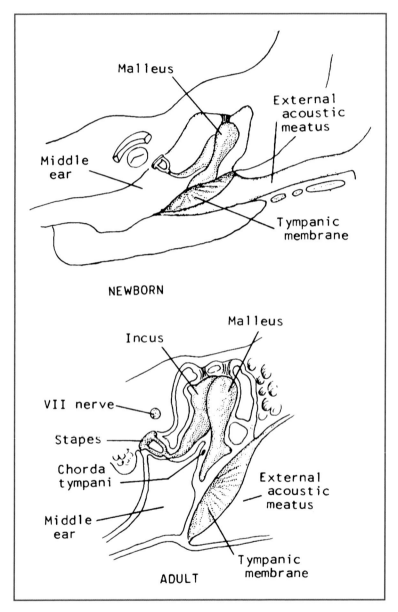

Figure 2–11. *Position of the tympanic membrane in the new born, and the adult. (Redrawn with permission from G. H. William. Developmental anatomy of the ear. In G. M. English [Ed.], 1988.* Otolaryngology, Vol. I, Diseases of the Ear and Hearing. *Rev. ed. Philadelphia, PA: J. B. Lippincott Company).*

Table 2–2. Chronology of the Embryonic Development of the Ear

Fetal Week	Inner Ear	Middle Ear	External Ear
3rd	Auditory placode: auditory pit	Tubotympanic recess begins to develop	
4th	Auditory vesicles (otocyst); vestibular-cochlear division		Tissue thickening begins to form
5th			Primary auditory meatus begins
6th	Utricle and saccule present; semicircular canals begin		Six hillocks evident; cartilage begins to form
7th	One cochlear coil present; sensory cells in utricle and saccule		Auricles move dorsolaterally
8th	Ductus reuniens present: sensory cells in semicircular canals	Incus and malleus present in cartilage; lower half of tympanic cavity formed	Outer cartilaginous third of external canal formed
9th		Three tissue layers at tympanic membrane are present	
11th	Two and one-half cochlear coils present; nerve VIII attaches to cochlear duct		
12th	Sensory cells in cochlea; membranous labyrinth complete; otic capsule begins to ossify		
15th		Cartilaginous stapes formed	

continues

Table 2–2. *continued*

Fetal Week	Inner Ear	Middle Ear	External Ear
16th		Ossification of malleus and incus begins	
18th		Stapes begins to ossify	
20th	Maturation of inner ear; ear adult size		Auricle adult shape but continues to mature until age 9
21st		Meatal plug disintegrates, exposing tympanic membrane	
30th		Pneumatization of tympanum	External auditory canal continues to mature until age 7
32nd		Malleus and incus complete ossification	
34th		Mastoid air cells develop	
35th		Antrum is pneumatized	
37th		Epitympanum is pneumatized; stapes continues to develop until adulthood; tympanic membrane changes relative position during first 2 years of life	

Source: Reproduced with permission from Northern and Downs, 1992. *Hearing in Children* (4th ed.). Baltimore, MD: Williams and Wilkins.

Structural Changes in the Elderly

The skin lining the ear canal undergoes changes similar skin in other parts of the body. Several important changes occur in the structure of the skin lining the ear canal as a result of aging. These changes with aging skin are: thinning of the surface epithelium and the atrophy of the subcutaneous tissue, reduced production oil by the sebaceous glands causing dryness and itchiness. Men experience a minimal decrease, usually after the age of 80, women gradually produce less oil beginning after menopause. This can make it harder to keep the skin moist and cerumen becomes more concentrated and often hard and impacted. In addition a slight rubbing or pulling on the skin can cause skin tears; fragile blood vessels can be easily broken. It is important to remember while performing cerumen extraction that older adults might be prone to bleeding and laceration of the skin. In addition, the hair follicles in the ear canal lose their elasticity and become stiff thereby obstructing the migration of cerumen that can lead to higher propensity of impaction in older adults.

3

Anatomy of the Ear Canal

RICHARD T. MIYAMOTO AND
R. CHRISTOPHER MIYAMOTO

A schematic view of the ear canal is shown in Figure 3–1. The skeletal structure of the ear canal consists of elastic cartilage laterally and bone medially. The narrowest portion of the ear canal or the isthmus is located just medial to the junction of the fibrocartilaginous and bony canals. The cartilage of the ear canal is continuous with that of the auricle. The cartilage of the tragus is in continuity with that of the auricle proper inferiorly. Anterosuperiorly, a gap exists between the cartilage of the helix and that of the tragus (tragohelicine incisure). Medially, the meatal cartilage is firmly attached to the bony meatus. The cartilaginous portion of the meatus constitutes approximately the outer one-third of the total length of the ear canal. In its anterior aspect, two or three inconstant, vertical fissures (Santorini fissures) filled with connective tissue pierce the cartilage. These fissures are a potential route for the spread of neoplasm or infections between the parotid gland and the external auditory canal. The cartilaginous is slightly concave anteriorly.

The medial one-third of the ear canal is osseous (Figure 3–1) and is oriented in a forward and downward direction. The bony meatus is slightly concave posteriorly so that the ear canal as a whole is slightly S-shaped. Because of the different angulations of the cartilaginous and bony canals, the adult auricle must be pulled upward and posteriorly to allow visualization of the tympanic membrane during otoscopic/ear canal examination. The anterior, inferior, and lower posterior parts of the bony wall of the ear canal are formed by the tympanic part of the temporal bone developed from the annulus tympanicus of the fetus. The

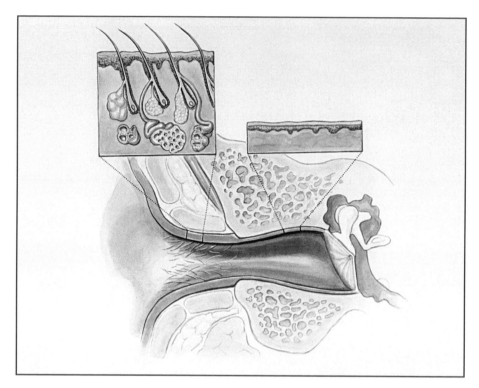

Figure 3–1. *Ear canal depicting the cartilaginous and osseous parts. Note the difference in the thickness of the skin lining the cartilaginous and bony areas. The secretory glands and the hair follicles are located in the cartilaginous portion of the canal. (Illustration by Sharon Tate. Medical Illustrations Department, Indiana University School of Medicine. Indianapolis, IN. Copyright 1994 Medical Illustrations Department of the Indiana University School of Medicine). Reproduced with permission.*

annulus remains incomplete posterosuperiorly. Therefore, the bony wall of the adult meatus is completed by the squamous and petrous parts of the temporal bone. In the infant, the bony canal is very short prior to the development of the annulus and mastoid process. The tympanic membrane is directed more inferiorly than laterally. In the adult, the tympanic membrane retains some of its downward and inward slope. The posterosuperior wall of the external canal measures approximately 25 mm in length, where as the anteroinferior wall is about 6 mm longer. The anterior and inferior walls of the meatus are closely related to the parotid gland. The anterior wall of the bony meatus is also closely related to the glenoid fossa and the condyle of the mandible.

The skin of the osseous canal is much thinner than that of the cartilaginous canal, measuring about 0.2 mm in thickness and is continuous with the skin covering the lateral surface of the tympanic membrane. No glands or hair follicles are found in the bony canal. The thickness of the skin of the bony ear canal predisposes this portion of the canal to trauma during manipulations such as removing cerumen. Thermal irritation of the periosteum of the bony canal may result from swimming in cold water, leading to the formation of bony growths or exostoses. The thin skin must also be accounted for during surgical procedures in the bony canal to prevent inadvertent laceration.

The skin of the fibrocartilaginous portion of the canal averages 0.5 to 1 mm in thickness. Many hair follicles are found in the lateral one-third of the fibrocartilaginous canal. Both modified apocrine (ceruminous) and sebaceous glands develop from the outer root sheath of the hair follicles, as shown in Figure 3–1.

Blood Supply

The auricle has an abundant blood supply from the posterior auricular artery and from small auricular branches of the superficial temporal artery. The vascular supply to the ear canal and the auricles is portrayed in Figure 3–2. The ear canal receives blood supply from the same vessels as the auricle, but also receives branches from the deep auricular artery, a branch from the first part of the internal maxillary artery. The deep auricular artery courses through the parotid gland and behind the capsule of the temporomandibular joint to penetrate either the bony or cartilaginous part of the meatus and supply the deeper part of the ear canal and the tympanic membrane.

The venous drainage from the auricle and meatus is through the superficial temporal and posterior auricular veins. The lymphatic drainage of the auricle and meatus join and empty into adjacent lymph nodes. Anteriorly, drainage is to the parotid nodes; inferiorly, drainage is to the superficial cervical nodes along the jugular vein; and posteriorly drainage is to the retroauricular nodes resulting in enlargement of these nodes. Therefore, confusion may arise between the diagnosis of external otitis and acute mastoiditis.

Innervation

Figure 3–3 depicts the sensory innervation of the auricle and the ear canal is supplied chiefly by branches of cranial nerves V, X, and the cervical plexus, but also receive branches from cranial nerves VII and IX.

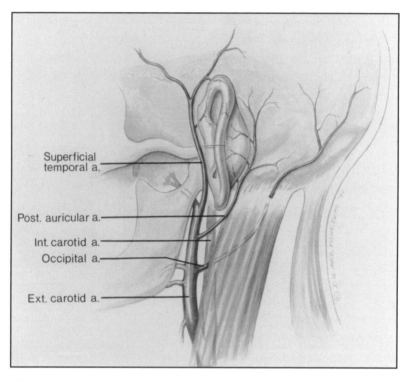

Superficial temporal a.

Post. auricular a.

Int. carotid a.

Occipital a.

Ext. carotid a.

Figure 3–2. *Blood supply to the pinna and the ear canal. (Illustration by Sharon Tate. Medical Illustrations Department, Indiana University School of Medicine. Indianapolis, IN. Copyright 1994 Medical Illustrations Department of the Indiana University School of Medicine). Reproduced with permission.*

Due to overlap of the areas of the auricle and ear canal innervated by these cutaneous nerves and natural variations, the precise distribution of these nerves is not constant. The approximate innervation of this region may be generalized as follows.

The auriculotemporal nerve (mandibular branch of cranial nerve V) supplies the anterior superior quadrant of the auricle, from the anterior part of the helix down to the tragus. Additionally, the auriculotemporal nerve innervates the anterior wall of the ear canal and anterior part of the external side of the tympanic membrane.

The great auricular nerve, originates from nerve C2 and C3 of the cervical plexus and supplies the majority of the posterior surface of the auricle: the helix, antihelix, and lobule. The superior medial part of the auricle is supplied by the lesser occipital nerve (originating from nerve C2 of the cervical plexus), which overlaps the area supplied by the greater auricular nerve.

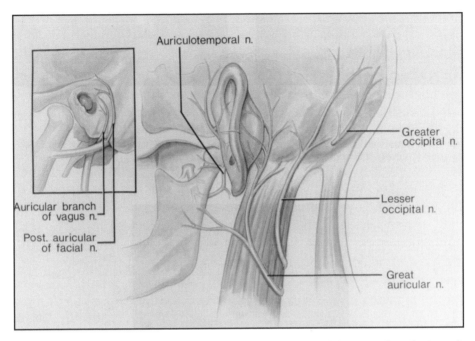

Figure 3–3. *Nerve supply to the pinna and the ear canal (ear canal in the insert). (Illustration by Sharon Tate. Medical Illustrations Department, Indiana University School of Medicine. Indianapolis, IN. Copyright 1994 Medical Illustrations Department of the Indiana University School of Medicine). Reproduced with permission.*

Cranial nerve X, with contributions from cranial nerves VII and IX, supplies the depression of the concha, posterior wall of the ear canal and the posterior portion of the external surface of the tympanic membrane.

Tympanic Membrane

The tympanic membrane (TM) separates the ear canal from the middle ear cavity. The tympanic membrane is approximately one cm in diameter and rests obliquely in the ear canal, with its outer surface facing outward, downward, and forward, forming a 55-degree angle with the floor of the ear canal (Woodburne, 1978). Laterally, the tympanic membrane is covered by thin skin continuous with that lining the ear canal. It is covered medially by mucosa of the middle ear cavity. Connective tissue exists between the lateral skin and medial mucosal layers. This connective tissue layer consists of a peripheral group of circular fibers surrounding a more numerous group of fibers radiating out from the manubrium of the malleus. These circular fibers form a fibrocartilaginous ring around the edge of the tympanic membrane, attaching the eardrum to the tympanic sulcus of the temporal bone. The tympanic sulcus is not complete at the superior edge of the tympanic membrane, nor are there connective tissue fibers. This portion of the tympanic membrane (one-sixth of the total area) lacks rigidity and is termed the pars flaccida. The remaining five-sixths of the tympanic membrane is termed pars tensa.

The eardrum is concave, with the center of the concavity formed by the attachment of the tympanic membrane to the manubrium of the malleus. This point of attachment is termed the umbo. The lateral process of the malleus attaches to the anterosuperior part of the TM, forming the mallear folds. These folds pass out to the cartilaginous ring of the tympanic membrane and form the division between the pars flaccida and the pars tensa. An important clinical observation is the "cone of light" seen upon otoscopic examination of the tympanic membrane. This is an area of reflected light downward and anterior from the umbo (Hollinshead, 1968).

Vessels and Nerves of the Tympanic Membrane

The blood supply and innervation of the tympanic membrane are divided into segments supplying the external and internal aspects of the membrane. The largest vessel supplying the external tympanic membrane is the manubrial artery. The vessel originates above the tympanic membrane and descends in a direction posterior to the manubrium and ends overlying it. The deep auricular branch of the auricular artery also forms a vascular ring around the outer edge of the eardrum. Small artery branches extend into the tympanic membrane from the deep auricular, making up the remaining blood supply to the external tympanic membrane. The inner surface of the tympanic membrane is supplied by branches of the maxillary artery (anterior tympanic branch) and posterior auricular artery (stylomastoid branch).

The external side of the tympanic membrane is supplied by the auriculotemporal branch of cranial nerves V and X, with contributions from cranial nerves VII and IX. The internal surface of the tympanic membrane is supplied by the tympanic plexus of cranial nerve IX. Nerve fibers supplying the eardrum follow the path of the manubrial artery. They originate posterosuperiorly to the tympanic membrane and descend toward the umbo, stopping posterior to the manubrium. The pars flaccida has a large nerve supply whereas the pars tensa has little innervation.

4

Ear Canal Examination

BOPANNA B. BALLACHANDA

Ear canal examination is an important aspect of audiology practice. Be it for diagnosis or for rehabilitation, visually inspecting the pinna, ear canal, and tympanic membrane aids in the identification of conditions that might subvert audiological test results or complicate audiological rehabilitation. The purpose of ear canal examination can be divided into the following five major areas.

Identifying Pathological Conditions of the Pinna and Ear Canal

Ear canal and pinna examination may identify conditions that require prompt attention from a medical practitioner or an otologist. As audiologists receive extensive training in the anatomy, physiology, and pathologies of the ear, they are able to detect many pathological conditions, such as abnormalities of the skin, fungal infections, neoplasm, and edema. The presence of such pathological conditions in the ear canal may not always produce abnormal audiometric findings on air and bone conduction tests. However, these conditions may contraindicate making an earmold impression, inhibit the audiologist from performing immittance testing, or cause discomfort while placing/inserting earphones. It should be *emphasized that the purpose of ear canal examination by an audiologist is not to diagnose an ear disease or recommend treatment, but to help identify outer ear pathologies/abnormalities and advise the patient to seek prompt medical attention, if necessary.*

Detecting Conditions That Can Alter Audiological Test Results

The major reason for ear canal examination by an audiologist is to detect conditions that might adversely influence the outcome of audiologic test results. For example, a collapsed ear canal can elevate air conduction thresholds and induce a conductive loss; also, impacted cerumen can cause alterations in many of the procedures in the audiology battery such as immittance measures. Hence, it is important to perform a visual inspection of the pinna and ear canal before beginning audiological evaluations.

Previously, audiologists contended that as long as there was an opening for the sound to reach the tympanic membrane, the test results were not affected by ear canal obstructions. Audiologists are now aware that basic and advanced audiological test procedures mandate an unobstructed ear canal. Therefore, *one of the purposes of ear canal examination is to identify pathologies and obstructions that can adversely affect or alter audiological test results.*

In certain individuals (older adults and young children), the ear canal can collapse as a result of earphone pressure during audiometry, causing an additional threshold shift of about 20 dB across the audiometric test frequencies (Ginsberg & White, 1986). A careful examination of the concha and tragus can identify this problem. One way to circumvent the problem of a collapsed ear canal is to use insert earphones instead of circumaural earphones. Should the audiologist decide to use insert earphones, ear canal inspection would help in choosing appropriate size tips.

An occluded ear canal not only produces variations in audibility, but can also alter the resonance properties of the ear canal (Chandler, 1964). Chandler (1964) investigated the effects of ear canal occlusion on hearing sensitivity for both air and bone conduction measures at octave frequencies between 125 and 8000 Hz, as shown in Figure 4–1. Approximately 80, 90, 95, 98, 99, and 100% occlusions of the total volume of the canal were achieved by placing progressively larger custom-made earmolds in the canal. The results of that study suggest that the changes in hearing

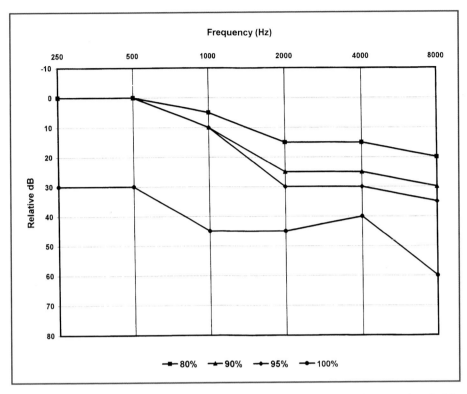

Figure 4–1. *Effect of ear canal occlusion on air and bone conduction thresholds. (Adapted from Chandler [1964]. Partial occlusion of the external acoustic meatus. Its effect upon air and bone conduction hearing acuity.* Laryngoscope, *22, 22–36.)*

sensitivity were a function of the type of stimuli used and the amount of blockage present; the air conduction thresholds were elevated significantly higher than the bone conduction thresholds. Threshold shifts of up to 40 dB were noted at frequencies greater than 1000 Hz when the occlusion was 80%; however, the lower frequencies were equally affected as the amount of occlusion increased from 80 to 100%. Therefore, *one of the reasons for ear canal examination is to identify ear canal occlusion due to cerumen or foreign bodies.* Such occlusions might alter the degree and type of hearing loss; for example a 40 dB pure sensory neural hearing loss may be identified as a mixed loss, or normal hearing might be misdiagnosed as a conductive loss.

During immittance measurements, pinna, ear canal, and tympanic membrane inspections can help determine the probe tip size; orientation of the probe so that the sound is directed toward the tympanic membrane; and contraindications for placement of the probe, such as cerumen impaction, laceration, and bleeding (Pearlman & Hoffman, 1976).

Another situation that requires a careful examination of the ear canal is during electrode placement in the canal for recording inner ear (ECochG) and auditory brainstem responses (ABR). The commercially available ear canal electrodes, for example, leaf electrodes (Coats, 1974), "Tiptrodes^R" and tympanic membrane electrodes or "Tymptrodes" (Cullen, Ellis, Berlin, & Lousteau, 1972; Stypulkowski & Staller, 1987), mandate clean ear canals to optimize recording conditions and electrode placement closer to the tympanic membrane. As a result, audiologists are frequently involved in examining the ear canal to ascertain that it is clean and open before placing electrodes.

Furthermore, otoacoustic emissions are routinely used in screening and diagnosis of inner ear problems in children and adults. In order to obtain otoacoustic emission (OAE) measurements, careful evaluation of the ear canal and proper placement of the probe in the canal is essential. Studies have shown that slight alterations in microphone placement can cause substantial variations in the sound level measured within the ear canal (Rabbitt & Friedrich, 1991).

Assessment of the ear canal and tympanic membrane (TM) is vital during caloric irrigation as part of the electronystagmography (ENG) test battery. *It is strongly recommended that caloric irrigation should be avoided in the presence of TM perforation, pressure equalization (PE) tubes, and ear canal pathologies to prevent possible damage to the middle and/or inner ear structures.*

Determining Need for Cerumen Management

The most common obstruction to visualizing the tympanic membrane is cerumen (Roland et al., 2008). Detection and management of cerumen depends on careful and thorough inspection of the pinna, ear canal, and tympanic membrane. Indeed, the presence of cerumen usually goes unnoticed until a visual inspection of the ear canal and tympanic membrane is performed (Gleitman, Ballachanda, & Goldstein, 1992).

Ear canal examination enables audiologists to gather information pertaining to type (dry or wet) and consistency (soft or hard) of the cerumen, the amount of blockage, and the necessity for softening. Ear canal examination should also provide information concerning the presence of contraindications for extracting cerumen and the need to implement universal precautions for blood and fluid-borne pathogens. Information gathered during *ear canal examination is also critical for deciding whether to proceed with cerumen management or to refer the patient to a medical facility. Ear canal examination is especially important during post extraction evaluation to determine the outcome of the procedure and status of the ear canal.*

Identifying Conditions That Mandate Implementation of Universal Blood and Fluid Precautions

Several epidemiological studies indicate that health care professionals, including audiologists, are at greater risk of contracting infectious diseases than are nonhealth care professionals (ASHA, 1989; 1990; Ballachanda 1994; Ballachanda, Roeser, & Kemp,1995; Kalcioglu et al., 2004; McMillan & Willette, 1988). Acquired immune deficiency syndrome (AIDS) has aroused great concern among audiologists and other health care professionals, prompting them to implement precautionary measures to prevent the spread of this disease to themselves, their families, and their patients (McMillan & Willette, 1988). Based on the Centers for Disease Control (CDC) recommendation that "blood and body fluids containing visible blood from all clients should be handled as though they were vehicles of the AIDS/HIV virus." During ear canal inspection audiologists must identify the presence of blood or bleeding in the canal. Although there are no clear indications to suggest that AIDS/HIV virus can be transmitted through cerumen (Sooy et al., 1987), it is conceivable that cerumen could be contaminated with blood. In such instances it is prudent to exercise universal precautions for blood and body fluid-borne pathogens. Similarly, the hepatitis B virus can only be transmitted by the body secretions and serum of infected people, which includes whom the disease has not been clinically diagnosed.

Kalcioglu et al. (2004) examined the cerumen samples collected from patients confirmed to have HBV DNA sera. It is reported that HBV-B virus affects almost 5% of the world's population amounting to 350 to 400 million persons. It is important for both otologists and audiologist, especially to audiologists, to implement precautionary measures to minimize the exposure to the disease. The findings from the Kalcioglu (2004) study suggest that HBV can be detected in cerumen like other fluids when the serum HBV DNA levels are high.

Identifying Conditions That Might Delay or Inhibit Nonmedical Rehabilitative Procedures

A thorough examination of the ear canal and tympanic membrane should always be made with an otoscope before taking an impression for earmolds, plugs, or hearing aids. Audiologists should study the ear canal and the earmold impression carefully to determine that the impression is a faithful replica of the ear canal (size and shape). An improper ear impression can lead to a poorly fitting hearing aid or earmold which may cause feedback and inadequate amplification that could have been avoided if a thorough inspection of the ear canal and the impression was performed before making the earmold. An understanding of ear canal anatomy combined with visual inspection can significantly reduce the number of hearing aids returned for shell modification or poor fit.

Visual inspection of the ear canal can also determine any restrictions to obtaining ear mold impressions (e.g., tympanic membrane perforation) and identify postsurgical indentations in the ear canal. Malformations that normally would be regarded as irregularities by hearing aid manufacturers or earmold laboratories should be noted on the order form. It is strongly recommended to inspect the ear canal for any materials that might have remained inside after the impression is pulled out of the canal.

Ear canal examination is equally important for probe microphone measurements. There are strong indications that results are often subject to error due to changes in the position of the microphone when measurements are repeated (Dirks & Kincaid, 1987).

Instrumentation

Ear canal examination can be carried out using several types of instruments. A major prerequisite for ear canal examination is adequate illumination of the canal. According to Hawke, Keene, and Alberti (1990), originally the ear canal examination was performed under sunlight; though it served the purpose, sunlight was not reliable during the winter months or on cloudy days. These concerns prompted clinicians to use artificial light. The quest for ever brighter artificial light has taken clinicians from candles to oil lamps and finally to present day fiberoptic and halogen lights (Hawke, Keene, & Alberti, 1990). The addition of magnifying lenses has enhanced our ability to visualize and assess the status of the ear canal and tympanic membrane more accurately.

There are several commercially available instruments routinely used for ear canal and tympanic membrane examination. The most commonly used instruments are described here.

Head Mirror

The head mirror is a circular concave mirror with a central aperture, mounted on a headband as shown in Figure 4–2. The mirror has a diameter of 3½" which is large enough to concentrate the light but small

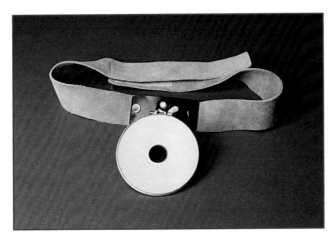

Figure 4–2. *Head mirrors are concave optical glass diameter 3½" with a central aperture of ¾". Headbands can be made of leather or plastic materials.*

enough not to obstruct the vision. The central aperture diameter is ¾" and is designed to permit visualization of the ear canal with the help of one eye. The mirror is mounted to a headband with a gooseneck joint, which permits the examiner to rotate or adjust the mirror to any angle and height. The headbands can be adjustable to fit any head size. A limitation of the head mirror is that it depends on an external light source; however, this limitation can be overcome by using any commercially available light source. A major advantage of the head mirror is that it frees both hands to insert instruments and perform procedures.

The Head Light

The head light, a recent invention, is worn on the center of the forehead as shown in Figure 4–3. The illumination in most head lights is provided by a halogen lamp; compared to other forms of illumination, halogen lamps are significantly brighter and more evenly distributed. In most head lights the focusing sleeve adjusts the beam to permit uniform illumination. The light bulb is mounted on the headband with a gooseneck joint, enabling the examiner to control the height and angle of the light beam.

Advantages of the head light are: illumination is even; the light source moves with the head of the examiner, thus providing better visualization; and freedom of both hands for instrumentation. A disadvantage is the absence of coaxial illumination; however, some manufacturers have overcome this problem by incorporating a perforated mirror for illumination and viewing.

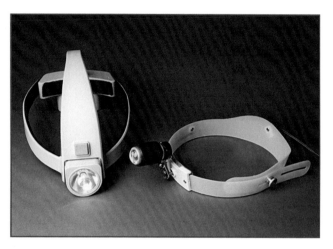

Figure 4–3. *Electric head lights.*

Otoscope

Otoscopes are the most popular instruments for examining the ear canal and tympanic membrane. They are hand held, and thus capable of delivering light into the deeper parts of the ear canal. A standard otoscope is made up of two parts, the head and the handle as shown in Figure 4–4. The light source and the viewing port are located on one side, which can be either cylindrical or oval in shape; the other side tapers off to produce an elongated narrow opening known as the nose. The specula, disposable or reusable, can be firmly attached to the nose during otoscopy. The beam produced by the light source, located within the head, is directed toward the nose into the canal. The examiner can visualize the structures in the ear canal by placing an eye near the viewing port.

Different head sizes serve specific purposes. For example, in the operating otoscope shown in Figure 4–5, a small rotatable magnifying lens is mounted slightly behind the lamp to provide additional magnification, while the head is completely open to insert instruments for otological procedures. In contrast, the pneumatic otoscope head, also shown in Figure 4–5, is closed on all sides except the opening in the nose. The specula fits snugly in the canal, and the air pressure within the ear canal can be altered by squeezing the rubber bulb of the insufflator attachment. In teaching otoscopes, there are two viewing ports for simultaneous visualization by the examiner and the observer.

The power source for the head in all otoscopes is supplied by disposable batteries, rechargeable cadmium batteries, or an AC transformer. The handle of the otoscope houses either disposable batteries (two AA

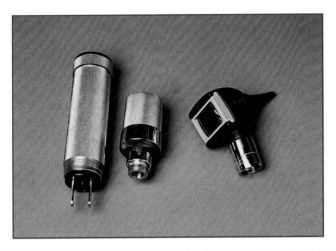

Figure 4–4. *Two parts of a standard otoscope; handle* (left side); *head* (right side).

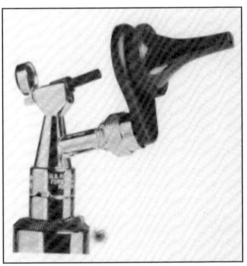

A

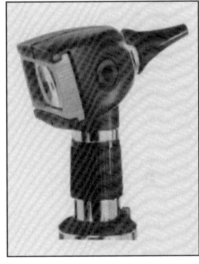

B

Figure 4–5. *Otoscope heads.* **A.** *Operating otoscope.* **B.** *Pneumatic otoscope.*

or C batteries) or a rechargeable cadmium battery; in some cases a rechargeable battery pack such as that shown in Figure 4–6 is preferable because, while the power of the disposable batteries decreases with use, the rechargeable battery pack provides uniform voltage until the power is completely used up. The AC powered otoscopes are light and the power source is constant; however, they are wall mounted and not portable (see Figure 4–6).

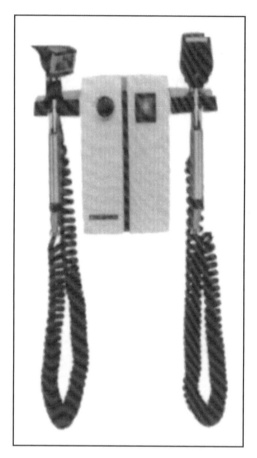

Figure 4–6. *Otoscope: wall mounted and not portable AC powered.*

Hotchkiss Otoscope

The Hotchkiss otoscope shown in Figure 4–7A was designed to permit unobstructed access for instrumentation and viewing under full magnification. This otoscope was developed by an otolaryngologist to combine the optical principles of the head mirror with features of the otoscope. The concave mirror optical system gathers the light rays produced by the xenon gas filled bulb and focuses them along the line of vision so that the area illuminated and the area viewed are the same. This coaxial optical system eliminates the parallax error that is usually present in conventional otoscopes. This design, developed over 12 years, enables clinicians to perform procedures, such as cerumen removal, inserting PE tubes, and even myringotomies, that once would have required an operating microscope. The Hotchkiss otoscope is designed to be held by the thumb and index finger of one hand as demonstrated in Figure 4–7B,

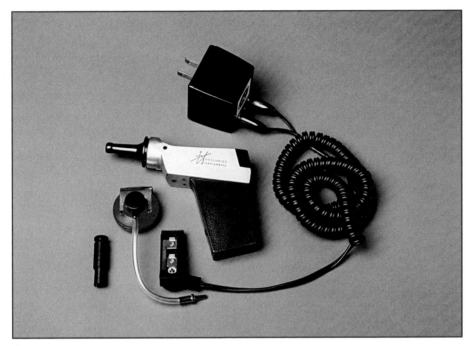

A

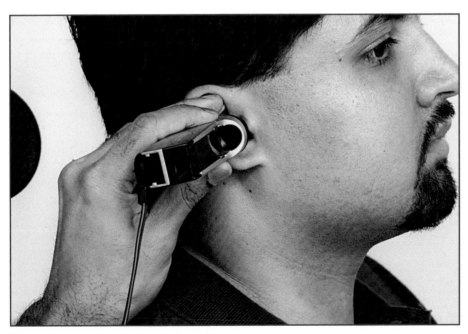

B

Figure 4–7. Hotchkiss otoscope. **A.** Battery pack, AC adapter, magnifying unit (×5), and the insufflator attachment. **B.** Held by the thumb and index finger of one hand for visualization of ear canal and the tympanic membrane. (Courtesy of Preferred Products.)

freeing the middle finger of the same hand for canal straightening. Thus, the other hand may be used for cerumen removal or insertion of instruments for other procedures.

Video-otoscope

The video-otoscope, shown in Figure 4–8, is a simple, compact unit that incorporates a rod system, fiberoptic illumination, and a high-resolution color video camera capable of recording images of patients' ear canals and tympanic membranes. By projecting the image on a video monitor, the video-otoscope enables the clinician to compare the ear canal and tympanic membrane before and after treatment, and allows patients and accompanying persons to see the ear canal and tympanic membrane during examination. The video-otoscope can be used to produce a permanent Polaroid-type photograph of the image or a video tape recording of it for documenting treatment procedures. Due to popular demands for video-otscopes, a variety of video-otoscopes have come in use in recent years. The most recent ones use a camera and the image is displayed on a

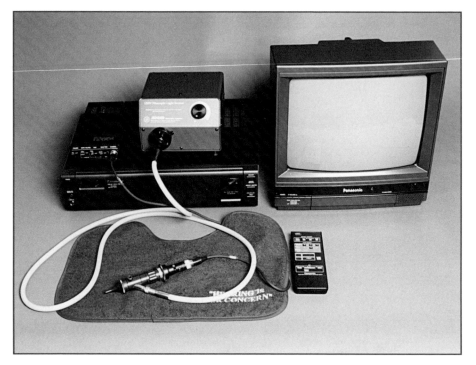

Figure 4–8. *Video-otoscope: TV monitor, S video recorder, probe unit with a camera and fibro-optic illumination unit, power supply. (Courtesy of Starkey Laboratories)*

computer monitor and stored as digital image in the computer. The price on these units has come down due to mass production and availability of high quality video cameras.

Surgical Loupe

Surgical loupes represent an innovative departure from the ordinary, unlike the surgical microscopes, learning to master the loupes is easy and only takes very minimal training (Figure 4–9). The main advantages to using loupes in the ear canal are: (1) hands-free: user has use of both hands, no longer required to tie up one hand holding the otoscope; (2) superior binocular, coaxial illumination and visualization—using both eyes for perfect depth perception, better magnification at 3.0×, and a much more powerful, brighter, whiter, shadow-free LED light system (with 6000 degree Kelvin temperature and anywhere from 20,000 to 50,000 Lux); and (3) working distance—advantageous working distance

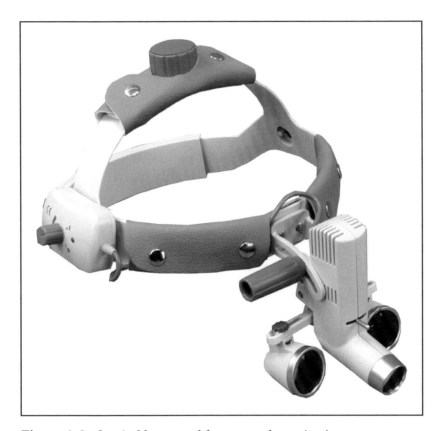

Figure 4–9. *Surgical loupe used for ear canal examination.*

of 340 mm (13.4°), the user no longer is required to hunch down peering through an otoscope within inches of the patients head, which is more comfortable for the user and the patient.

Loupes have rapidly become a preferred way of examining the ear canal by audiologists and otologists. It is critical that the loupes portray an accurate, precise, distortion-free view. With the flood of inexpensive and inferior quality loupes on the market, many professionals are confused. Loupes may look identical but have varying degrees of optical quality and clarity. Figure 4–10A is the original view by the naked eye, Figure 4–10B shows the view through inferior-quality loupes, and Figure 4–10C shows the view through high-quality loupes.

The most common signs of poor quality loupes are *low resolution, chromatic aberration,* and *spherical aberration*:

> *Resolution* is defined as an optical system's ability to form distinguishable images of objects separated by small distances and the ability to recognize fine detail. This is a must in medical, dental, and veterinarian sciences.

> *Chromatic aberration* refers to color distortion. Because each color has a different wavelength, uncorrected optics cause the various wavelengths to focus at different points in space. The first color to fall out of focus is blue. Notice the blue haze just to the side of the black lines in Figure 4–10B. Tissue and color rendition is critical for any practitioner.

> *Spherical aberration* refers to the image's flatness. When viewed **through** loupes, an object that exhibits spherical aberrations would appear to be curved or spherical also depicted in Figure 4–10B. Distortions of any kind are unacceptable especially in tight areas such as the ear canal.

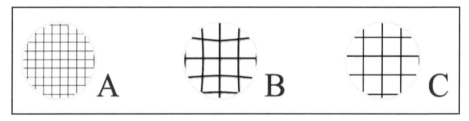

Figure 4–10. *Surgical loupe: varying degrees of optical quality and clarity.* **A.** *The original view by the naked eye.* **B.** *The view through inferior-quality loupes.* **C.** *The view through high-quality loupes.*

Operating Microscope

Microscopes, like that shown in Figure 4–11, represent the state-of-the-art visualization of the tympanic membrane and the ear canal because they provide a three-dimensional view, free both hands, and offer variable amounts of magnification. Although microscopes are primarily

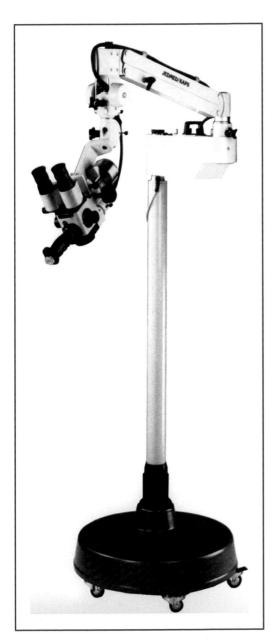

Figure 4–11. *Operating microscope—floor stand model.*

used for surgery, they are also very useful diagnostic tools in audiology practice. There are various types of surgical operating microscopes that are used for different applications. One common type of operation microscope is used by ENT (ear, nose, and throat) physicians is adequate for audiology clinics. The binocular head of the microscope is straight without any angle and the focal length can be changed by using different lens under the head, which also changes the overall magnification. Most microscopes for surgery have motorized foot controls for at least the focusing of the image to free up hands to hold tools. The higher grade equipment has additional foot controls for movement of the head. Some motorized controls are located on the head assembly itself to control rotation of the head in multiple degrees of rotation as well as centering the optics on the area of interest. An optional accessory on a surgical operating microscope is the use of video display. A system can be fitted with a beam splitter and C-mount for connection to a CCD color video camera. This type of microscope camera will output a composite video signal to a CCTV video monitor for viewing by others. Another optional accessory is the supplemental viewing ports that can be attached to the microscope to enhance its ability for multiple viewing. A significant factor to consider when purchasing a surgical operation microscope is the quality of the equipment and certifications held by the manufacturer. As this equipment is to be used in a medical/clinical setting, many countries require certification or registration of the equipment or manufacturing facility. In the United States, the U.S. Food and Drug Administration (US FDA) registers manufacturing facilities that make medical products. If the equipment you need is for a U.S. location, then you need one of our surgical microscopes that is made in an FDA-registered manufacturing facility.

Surgical microsopes are making inroad to audiology practice to accommodate a better visualization of the ear canal and placement of hearing aids into deeper parts of the ear canal. A number of audiologists are using surgical microscopes for visualization of the ear canal in order to place otoblocks for deep canal impressions as well as extended stay hearing aids in the canal.

Aural Specula

The aural speculum depicted in Figure 4–12 can be metal or plastic, reusable or disposable, but the inner surface must be nonreflective. Specula come in different sizes (between 2 mm and 5 mm in diameter). It is necessary to use the largest size appropriate for the ear canal being examined

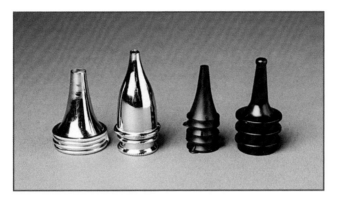

Figure 4–12. *Aural specula: metallic (left two sets) and plastic (right two sets).*

to permit visualization of the tympanic membrane as well as the insertion of instruments, if needed. Some practitioners hold the speculum by hand; others prefer to attach it to the otoscope.

Ear Canal Inspection

A careful visual inspection of the pinna and postauricular skin is important to detect tenderness, abnormalities, surgical scars, discharge, and skin disorders (Figure 4–13). In addition, inspection of the concha should reveal presence of excessive hair follicles and guide the clinician in selecting a speculum that fits in the patient's ear canal.

The patient should be seated comfortably in a chair, preferably an examination chair; a prototype is shown in Figure 4–14. The height of the chair should be adjusted such that the patient's ear canal and the examiner's eye are at the same level. As the canal is an S-shaped tube, it is difficult to visualize its deeper areas. To overcome this limitation, the canal can be straightened by pulling the pinna upward and backward in adults and horizontally backward in children. It is necessary to use a speculum that fits comfortably at the entrance of the canal to provide optimal visualization of the cartilaginous and bony parts of the ear canal as well as the tympanic membrane. A small speculum in a large canal can create two problems: (a) it may not provide adequate visualization of the tympanic membrane, and (b) it may be inserted deep in the canal, thereby causing discomfort to the patient. In contrast, a large speculum in a small canal may be uncomfortable to the patient and distort the view of the ear canal.

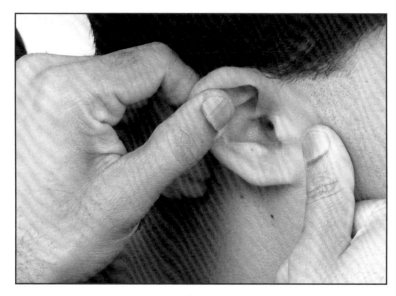

Figure 4–13. *Inspecting the entrance of the ear canal and the pinna. The pinna is retracted posterosuperiorly in the left hand to straighten the canal.*

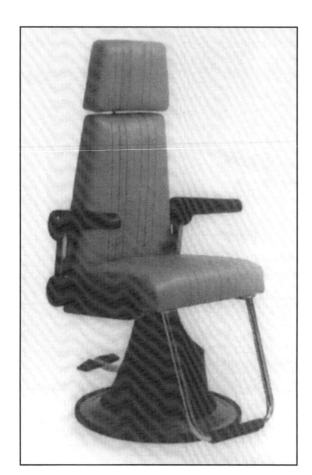

Figure 4–14. *Exam chair.*

There is no set procedure for holding an otoscope. One can hold it like a pencil as shown in Figure 4–15, or one can grip the scope at the top of the handle close to the light source as in Figure 4–16. If the otoscope is held as shown in Figure 4–15, then the fingers or the heel of the hand should be rested against the patient's temple. If the otoscope is held at

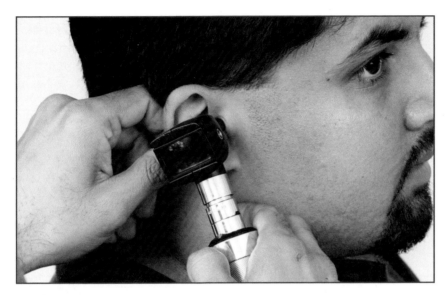

Figure 4–15. *Otoscope held as a pencil and the proper procedure to inspect the ear canal.*

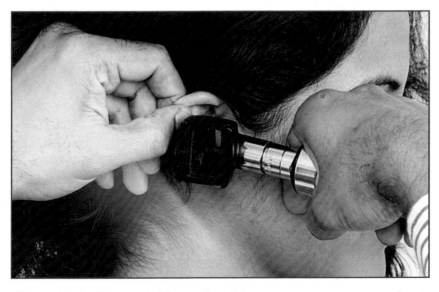

Figure 4–16. *Otoscope held near the light source and the proper procedure to inspect the ear canal.*

the top, similar to the way shown in Figure 4–16, the hand should be rested against the patient's cheek. These two anchoring procedures will help prevent the speculum from being accidentally inserted deep into the canal in case of sudden head movement. Figure 4–17 illustrates the correct way to hold the otoscope; it should be held close to the light source rather than at the bottom of the handle which can lead to poor visualization and a greater risk of damaging the ear canal.

The examiner's eye (one eye, not two, while using otoscopes) should be about an inch from the viewing port/magnifying glass. Occasionally, the examiner may need to adjust the speculum or the patient's head to obtain a clearer and better view of the ear canal and the tympanic membrane.

Once a clear view of the ear canal and the tympanic membrane is established, the examiner should probe and document the following conditions: (a) color, size, and shape of the canal; (b) presence of excessive hair follicles, infections, bleeding, scars, foreign bodies, or cerumen in the canal; (c) any malformations of the ear canal worthy of noting in the patient's history/chart; (d) color of the tympanic membrane which

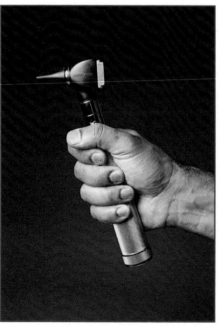 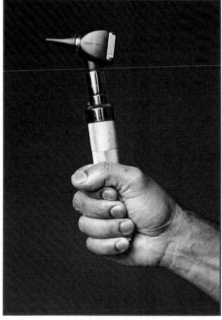

A   B

Figure 4–17. *Correct manner to hold the otoscope: should be held close to the light source as shown on the left side (**A**) and not like the figure on the right side (**B**).*

normally is pearly gray, and semitransparent; (e) visibility of the cone of light, head of the malleus and umbo, as shown in Figure 4–18; and (f) in addition, the shape of the tympanic membrane (i.e., retracted—negative pressure, or bulged out—fluid behind the tympanic membrane, would be worth noting during the examination).

If the object blocking the ear canal is cerumen, then the examiner should: (a) assess the type of cerumen (hard or soft) and the amount of blockage, (b) determine the necessity for cerumen softening, (c) resolve any questions on contraindications (see Chapter 9), and (d) determine the appropriate procedure(s) to extract the cerumen. Of course, the examiner should always remember to implement universal precautions for blood and body fluid borne pathogens.

In summary, it is worthwhile for audiologists to perform ear canal examination to avoid complications and obtain reliable test results from patients. A thorough understanding of the anatomy and pathologies of the ear canal, and the trained use of an appropriate light source, can enable audiologists to make accurate evaluations of ear canal pathologies and other problems.

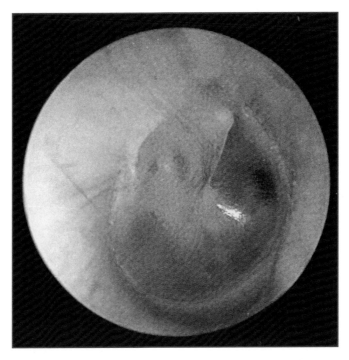

Figure 4–18. *Normal tympanic membrane. Notice the cone of light and end of the long process of the incus.*

5

Ear Canal Pathology

**RICHARD T. MIYAMOTO AND
R. CHRISTOPHER MIYAMOTO**

Pathological conditions of the ear canal may be of congenital, infectious, traumatic, or neoplastic origin.

Congenital Abnormalities

Congenital abnormalities of the external auditory canal occur in mild to severe forms and may range from mild stenosis to complete atresia. The continuum of deformities that can occur with congenital atresia of the ear are the result of arrested development of the bony or cartilaginous portion of the canal at any point in the embryologic process. This condition may be seen with or without significant pinna abnormalities or in association with other congenital craniofacial anomalies (Figure 5–1).

The external ear develops from the upper end of the first and second branchial arches and from the upper end of the first branchial cleft. The auricle develops from the six hillocks situated around the primitive meatus. The hillock that develops into the tragus is derived from the second branchial arch whereas the other five hillocks arise from the first branchial arch. By the end of the third month, the primitive auricle has completed its development.

During the second embryonic month, a solid core of epithelium migrates inward from the rudimentary pinna toward the first branchial pouch. This epithelial core is the precursor of the ear canal. The first branchial pouch grows outward to form the middle ear cleft. The interface

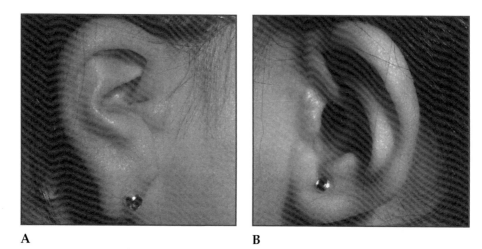

A   B

Figure 5–1. **A.** *Atresia of the ear canal. Pinna is minimally affected.* **B.** *Left normal ear canal and the pinna for the same patient shown in* A.

between the first branchial cleft and the first branchial pouch forms the tympanic membrane. During the sixth month, the epithelial core begins to hollow out and canalize from its medial end. Arrested or incomplete canalization results in varying degrees of stenosis or complete atresia.

Abnormalities of ear canal development may occur in association with numerous syndromes. For example, children with Down syndrome commonly have stenotic ear canal. This may predispose the patient to blockage from cerumen and debris and may result in conductive hearing loss. The Treacher-Collin syndrome is a congenital, first and second branchial arch syndrome displaying atresia of the ear canal in addition to hypoplasia of the maxilla and mandible. The presence of one congenital anomaly increases the probability of a second congenital abnormality, such as malformation or fixation of the middle ear ossicles. In selected cases, the conductive hearing loss associated with an atretic ear canal can be addressed by surgically creating a patent channel to the middle ear. The associated tympanic membrane and ossicular abnormalities are addressed using standard tympanoplasty technique.

Stenosis, or narrowing, of the ear canal may also occur on a congenital basis but may also result from trauma or from inflammatory disease.

Infections

Otitis external, shown in Figure 5–2, is an infection of the lining epithelium of the ear canal. It is most commonly caused by a bacterial infection,

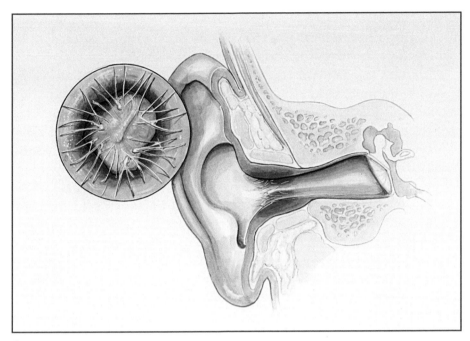

A

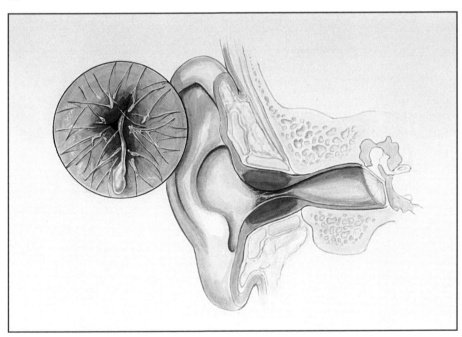

B

Figure 5–2. *Otis externa.* **A.** *Acute otitis externa. Note the red swollen ear canal skin and normal tympanic membrane.* **B.** *Acute otitis externa. Note the matkedly swollen ear canal skin and purulent drainage. (Illustration by Sharon Tate. Medical Illustrations Department, Indiana University School of Medicine. Indianapolis, IN. Copyright 1994 Medical Illustrations Department of the Indiana University School of Medicine). Reproduced with permission.*

but may result from fungal or viral agents. Symptoms of external otitis include pain which may be severe, itching, and sometimes fever.

Acute otitis externa is a bacterial infection of the ear canal caused by a break in the normal skin and cerumen protective barrier. This condition is commonly known as "swimmer's ear" but may be caused by anything that results in the removal of the protective lipid film from the canal allowing bacteria to enter the apopilosebaceous units. The warm, dark, moist environment present in the ear canal provides a perfect medium for rapid bacterial growth. Pain ensues as the swollen soft tissues of the canal distract the periosteal lining of the bony canal. With further progression of the disease, purulent discharge begins.

In patients in whom otitis externa is not resolved in the acute stage, a subacute or chronic form may occur. A spectrum of disease ranging form mild drying and scaling of the ear canal skin to complete obliteration of the canal by chronically infected and hypertrophic skin.

The usual pathogens responsible for acute otitis externa are *Pseudomonas aeruginosa*, staphylococci, *Proteus mirabilis*, streptococci, and various gram-negative bacilli.

Otomycosis

Otomycosis is a fungal infection of the skin of the ear canal (Figure 5–3). Fungi are usually superimposed on an uncontrolled, chronic bacterial infection of the ear canal or middle ear. Infrequently, otomycosis may occur as a primary infection.

Aspergillus species are the most common fungal pathogens. Pruritus is the primary clinical manifestation. Physical examination commonly shows a black, white, or dotted gray membrane. The matted fungal debris must be carefully removed and an acidifying solution, such as aluminum sulfate–calcium acetate (Domeboro), applied.

Malignant (Necrotizing) Otitis Externa

Malignant (necrotizing) otitis externa is a progressive necrotizing *Pseudomonas* infection of the ear. This condition should be suspected in any elderly, diabetic person who develops a persistent, painful external otitis. Poor control of diabetes mellitus is the most significant predisposing

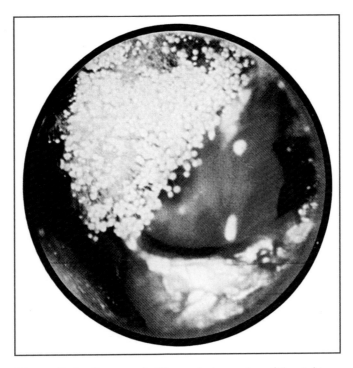

Figure 5–3. *Otomycosis. The posterior region of the right ear canal is filled with greenish-yellow fungus. (Reproduced with permission from* Atlas of Ear, Nose, and Throat Diseases *by W. Becker, R. A. Buckingham, P. H. Hollinger, W. Steiner, M. P. Jaumann, W Messerklinger, and W. Becker, 1984, p. 17. Copyright 1984 George Thieme Verlag, Stuttgart, Germany.)*

factor. Otalgia in this condition is generally more severe than in uncomplicated swimmer's ear and is typically most severe at night. Examination of the ear demonstrates the usual features of skin inflammation with redness, swelling, and tenderness. A classic feature of the malignant external otitis, seen in Figure 5–4, is the nubbin of granulation tissue found on the floor of the ear canal. This tissue arises at the junction of the bony and cartilaginous canal and is the result of osteitis of the lateral lip of the tympanic bone. Deeper tissues may be invaded in this area or initial invasion may occur through the fissures of Santorini.

At a later stage, infection may extend posteriorly to the stylomastoid foramen resulting in facial paralysis. If unchecked, the infection can spread up the facial canal into the mastoid. Further progression may lead to osteitis of the skull base and multiple cranial nerve palsies. Without intense treatment, skull base osteitis carries a high mortality rate.

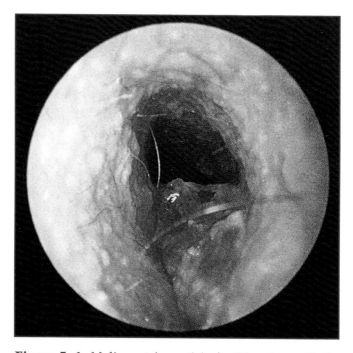

Figure 5–4. *Malignant (necrotizing) otitis externa. Fleshy granulation tissue arising in the canal. The disease process may spread to base of the skull, producing osteomyelitis of the temporal bone. (Reproduced with permission from* Diseases of the Ear: Clinical and Pathological Aspects *by M. Hawke and A. F. Jahn, 1987, p. 2.32. Copyright 1987 by Lea & Febiger.)*

There are three aspects to the treatment of malignant external otitis: First, and the most important aspect of therapy, is gaining control of the patient's diabetes mellitus. Second, the granulations are treated by local debridement. Third, systemic antibiotics must be administered in adequate amounts and for a long enough time. The usual antibiotics include an aminoglycoside and semisynthetic penicillin. Topical gentamicin and acetic acid preparation may be applied to the ear canal.

Trauma and Foreign Bodies

The lodgment of foreign bodies in the ear canal is a common pathology, especially in children (Figure 5–5). Swelling at the junction between the osseous and cartilaginous portion of the ear canal may occur if the object

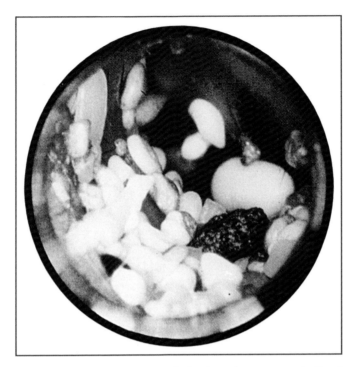

Figure 5–5. *Foreign body lodged in the ear canal. Coral and sand collected after surfing in the sea. (Reproduced with permission from* Atlas of Ear, Nose, and Throat Diseases *by W. Becker, R. A. Buckingham, P. H. Hollinger, W. Steiner, M. P. Jaumann, W. Messerklinger, and W. Becker, 1984, p. 17. Copyright 1984 George Thieme Verlag, Stuttgart, Germany.)*

is forced past this point. Vegetable matter, such as beans and seeds, pose an additional challenge because they tend to swell in the moist environment provided by the ear canal. Significant pain may result, as well as conductive hearing loss from the canal occlusion.

Cerumen (earwax) serves a protective function for the epithelial lining of the ear canal. It is normally cleared from the ear canal by epithelial migration. However, when excessively large amounts of cerumen are produced or the epithelial migration is inadequate, cerumen may become impacted into the ear canal. Hearing may not be affected by large amounts of cerumen as long as a communication remains between the external environment and the tympanic membrane. If the ear canal is completely occluded, a significant hearing loss may result. Care must be exercised when removing impacted cerumen to avoid abrading the delicate canal skin, especially in the bony ear canal.

Neoplasms

The ear canal may be the site of benign, premalignant, or malignant neoplastic changes in any of its structures including skin, glands, cartilage, bone, muscle, vessels, and nerves.

Keratosis Obturans

Keratosis obturans is a rare condition in which a keratotic mass of desquamating epithelium forms in the ear canal. If the impacted mass is not removed, there is ulceration of the skin and progressive erosion and enlargement of the osseous ear canal.

Exostosis and Osteoma

Exostoses are periosteal outgrowths which occur in the osseous canal of individuals who have done a great deal of swimming in cold water or whose ear canals have been exposed to other forms of trauma. As shown in Figure 5–6A, they are smooth, rounded, broad-based nodules adjacent to the annuls. They are usually bilateral and are more common in males than females. Removal is indicated only when they are large enough to obstruct the ear canal. In contrast, an osteoma (Figure 5–6B) occurs as a single benign tumor which resembles cortical bone. It occurs at the tympanomastoid suture line and tends to have a narrow base. As it grows it may cause recurrent entrapment of cerumen. Removal of an osteoma is frequently indicated.

Squamous Cell Carcinoma

Squamous cell carcinoma of the ear canal may initially appear as an ulcer, polyp, or subcutaneous mass. The lesions tend to grow slowly and if obstruction of the canal or infection occurs, the pain and drainage may simulate a chronic infection. Early biopsy of any suspicious lesion is advised.

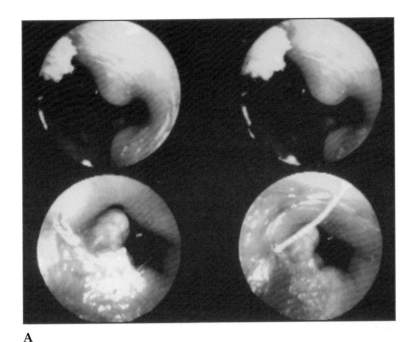

A

B

Figure 5–6. A. *Exotosis, due to swimming.* Top: *A large exotosis in the right ear that obstructs the view of the tympanic membrane.* Bottom: *A small exotosis in the left ear of the same patient.* **B.** *Osteoma.* Left: *Occupying the entire ear canal lumen.* Middle: *Specimen removed from the ear.* Right: *postsurgical. (Reproduced with permission from* Diseases of the Ear: Clinical and Pathological Aspects *by M. Hawke and A. F. Jahn, 1987, p. 2. Copyright 1987 by Lea & Febiger.)*

The tumor spreads the length of the canal and may invade the middle ear and extend into the mastoid, parotid gland, periauricular soft tissues and other contiguous structures. Metastases to regional lymph nodes occur slowly with the preauricular nodes generally involved first (Figure 5–7).

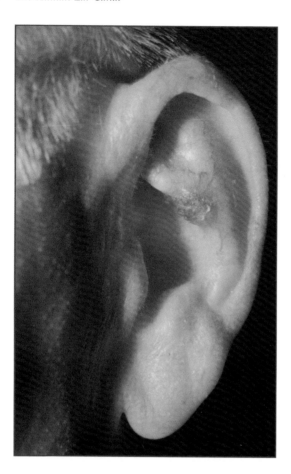

Figure 5–7. *A red pearly nodule is present adjacent to the antehelix. A biopsy demonstrates basal cell carcinoma. (Courtesy of C. William Hanke, MD).*

Basal Cell Carcinoma

Basal cell carcinoma of the ear canal is far less common than squamous cell carcinoma of the ear canal. Because of the tendency of this tumor to extend beyond the skin of the ear canal the prognosis is poor.

EAR CANAL CHOLESTEATOMA

Cholesteatoma are more common in the middle ear and mastoid, however, occasionally the disease process can spread to the ear canal in older adults. The ear canal cholesteatoma can be easily mistaken for keratosis obturans, the differentiating factor being that cholesteatoma is a localized invasive and destructive process as shown in Figure 5–8. Holt (1992) listed

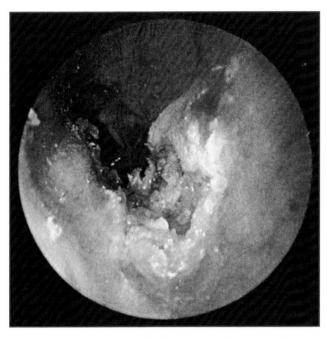

Figure 5–8. *Ear canal cholesteatoma. Due to cholesteatoma the bone is exposed in the inferior wall of the canal. (Reproduced with permission from* Diseases of the Ear: Clinical and Pathological Aspects *by M. Hawke and A. F. Jahn, 1987, p. 2.40. Copyright 1987 by Lea & Febiger).*

five possible etiology of cholesteatoma: they are postsurgical, posttraumatic, or due to ear canal stenosis, ear canal obstruction, or spontaneous.

Treatment options are: (a) frequent cleaning and application of mineral oil when the lesion is localized and small; (b) canaloplasty for deeper pockets either through transcanal or postauricular approach; and (c) mastoid surgery (Anthony & Anthony, 1982).

Tumors of Ceruminous Glands

Ceruminoma or tumor of the ceruminous glands either benign or malignant has been reported in clinical literature (Lynde, McLean, & Woods, 1984). The symptoms are variable: progressive hearing loss, discharge, and deep-seated pain may occur. The duration can also vary from a few months to several years. The tumor may be a polypoid mass in the ear canal or a large tumor extending into preauricular space; as the tumor enlarges erosion can occur.

6

Ear Canal Acoustics

BOPANNA B. BALLACHANDA

Introduction

The role of the outer ear (pinna and the ear canal) is to couple airborne sound waves to the middle ear. Understanding the functions of the outer ear requires an appreciation of basic acoustics and the process of transformation from the free-field or the earphone to the tympanic membrane. In the past several years there has been a considerable interest in specifying the dimensions of the outer ear to explain accurately the acoustic characteristics. A better understanding has emerged from increased reliance on measurements made within the ear canal for hearing aid prescription, earphone calibration, immittance measurements, high frequency audiometry, otoacoustic emission (OAE) measurements, and auditory brainstem response (ABR) testing and head-related transfer function (HRTF).

This chapter aims to provide a descriptive analysis of ear canal transfer functions from free-field to tympanic membrane with little reliance on mathematics beyond simple algebra. Topics discussed include: techniques to measure ear canal geometry; contributions of pinna and ear canal to sound pressure transformation from free-field to tympanic membrane; variables that can alter the pressure transformation within the ear canal; currently available outer ear simulators for acoustic measurements; and the importance of ear canal acoustics in audiology practice.

The materials covered are directed to hearing health professionals; it would have been more ambitious to review all the information on ear canal acoustics from the viewpoint of a physicist or a mathematician. Nevertheless, for scholarly review on ear canal acoustics, the reader is referred to the scientific articles cited in the reference section.

Techniques to Measure Ear Canal Geometry

The importance of ear canal geometry was recognized as early as 1882 by Bezold. Smelt, Hawke, and Proops (1988), in a review of earlier studies, indicated that Bezold (1882) made ear canal impressions of cadavers to determine the dimensions of the ear canal. Historically, the primary reason for obtaining ear canal impressions was to define the anatomic boundaries and to describe the relationship between the ear canal and the tympanic membrane. Even Helmholtz, as early as 1872, obtained ear-molds to describe the dimensions of the ear canal and the shape of the eardrum head.

The reported geometry of the ear canal includes the length of the canal at superior, middle, and inferior quadrants; the diameter of the canal; the area along the length of the canal; the total volume of the ear canal; and the angle of termination of the canal with respect to the tympanic membrane.

A variety of techniques have been used to measure ear canal geometry and the techniques have been refined over the years. The simplest method is to fill the canal with fluid (usually alcohol) to determine the volume and inserting a measuring gauge into the canal and progressing until it touched the tympanic membrane (Morton & Jones, 1956; Zwislocki, 1971) to measure the length. These measurements (i.e., the length and the total volume) were the only dimensions of importance to early researchers.

In quest for a better understanding of the dimensions, studies endeavored to obtain more detailed descriptions of the ear canal. Recent and more sophisticated procedures include precise physical measurements from ear canal impressions, to radiological techniques (i.e., computer-assisted tomography [CAT] or CT scanning), to mathematical computations based on sound pressure measurements at various locations within the canal (acoustic method), to clinical immittance measurements (impedance and reflectance), and recently the laser technology to scan the surface of the canal area/dimensions.

Physical Measurement

The earliest technique to measure the physical dimensions of the ear canal involved obtaining ear canal impressions, most often from cadaver ears, and subsequently from these impression or the cast of the impression physical dimensions were measured using various techniques. Johansen (1975) obtained 10 impressions of the entire ear canal (i.e., cartilaginous, bony parts) and the tympanic membrane from 10 cadavers (6 males and 4 females). The purpose of his study was to determine the volume of the ear canal as a function of the distance along the length of the canal from the tympanic membrane to the concha. The technique involved immersing the mold in a calibrated syringe containing 60% alcohol and measuring the fluid displacement at every 2 mm of immersion. He concluded that the volume of the adult ear was 101.4×10^{-2} cm^3 (±15.4 cm^3), and the mean length of the ear canal measured from the tympanic membrane to the cavum concha was 25.7 mm (±1.9 mm).

The current knowledge of the human ear canal geometry is quite complicated. Most importantly, the ear canal is not straight. It is rather tapered along its length. The canal is wider at the entrance where it flares out into the concha. The inner 10 mm of the canal forms a wedge-shaped cavity, with the eardrum forming the one side of the wedge. The ear canal contains twists and turns; it bends upward at the canal-concha junction, and then turns downward near the tympanic membrane. To support the fact that the ear canal is not a straight tube, a scanned image of the ear canal is shown in Figure 6–1. It is quite apparent that the canal is not straight and the total area function varies from the entrance of the canal to the second bend of the S-shaped canal. The canal dimensions vary considerably between individuals. According to Shaw (1974b) and others, these dimensions are very important when considering the effects on sound pressure distribution within the ear canal.

Stinson and Lawton (1989, p. 2492) indicated that "if quantitative predictions of the sound field in a real ear canal are desired, particularly at high frequencies, the uniform tube approximation must be abandoned" (Figure 6–2C). Up to this point the ear canal was approximated as a uniform tube; this representation provided a good approximation of pressure distribution up to 8.0 kHz. However, ability to predict the sound pressure level within the canal at higher frequencies required a better definition of the ear canal geometry. To accommodate the dimensional variations across and within subjects they suggested that the ear canal geometry be specified in relation to the curved axis as shown in Figure 6–2A, rather than the straight axis used by Hudde (1983) and

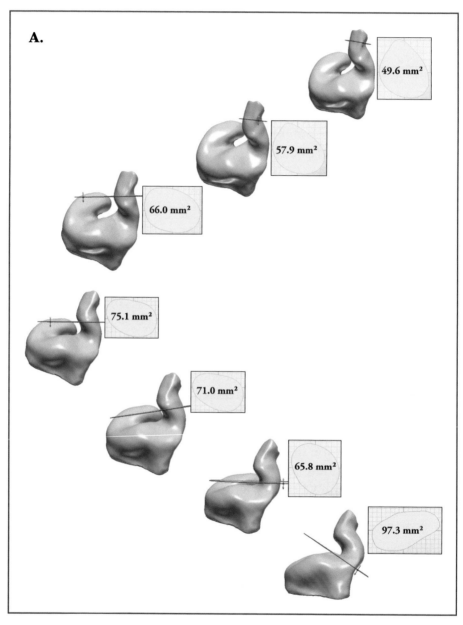

Figure 6–1. *Scanned image of the earmold taken from a subject. The area measurement is shown next to the circled lines. The area function varies at various locations along length of the canal from the entrance to the second bend. (Scanning provided by Starkey Laboratories, Eden Praire, MN)* continues

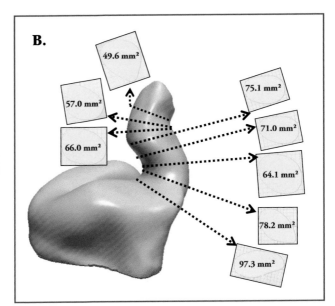

B.

49.6 mm²

57.0 mm²

66.0 mm²

75.1 mm²

71.0 mm²

64.1 mm²

78.2 mm²

97.3 mm²

Figure 6–1. continued

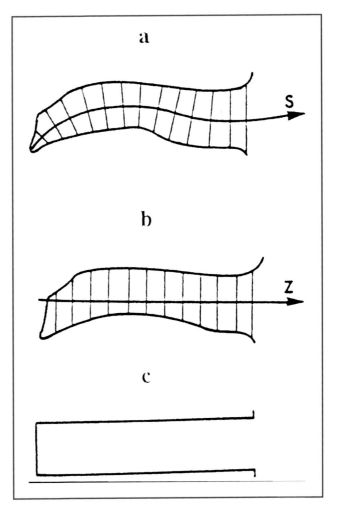

Figure 6–2. **A.** *The ear canal dimensions indicating the curved axis along the length of the ear canal and slices of varying cross-sectional areas.* **B.** *Uniform parallel slices with a straight axis.* **C.** *Uniform tube. (Adapted from Specification of the Geometry of the Human Ear Canal for the Prediction of Sound Pressure Level Distribution: M. R. Stinson and B. W. Lawton, 1989, p. 2493.* Journal of the Acoustical Society of America, 85. *Copyright 1989 American Institute of Physics)*

a

S

b

Z

c

several other researchers as shown in Figure 6–2B. This led to a detailed investigation by Stinson and Lawton (1989) to define the geometry of the canal using ear canal impressions and direct physical measurements of the dimensions. They obtained a total of 15 ear impressions from right and left cadaver ears. From these molds, utilizing a specialized mechanical probe system developed by the authors, approximately 1,000 points were measured over the entire surface of the mold, starting at the ear canal tympanic membrane junction and progressing toward the concha. The three-dimensional representation of these data points is shown in Figure 6–3. Using a computer program, three-dimensional models were developed and subsequently, the cross-sectional area along the curved central axis was measured.

They also noted that there were considerable variations in the canal size and shape across the subjects. The grouped data of the ear canal

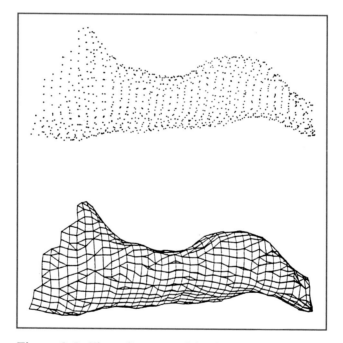

Figure 6–3. *Three-dimensional display of the geometry of the ear canal from 978 coordinate points measured from the earmold impression. The longitudinal cross-section reflects the parallel slices at 1 mm apart. (Reproduced with permission from Specification of the Geometry of the Human Ear Canal for the Prediction of Sound Pressure Level Distribution: M. R. Stinson and B. W. Lawton, 1989, p. 2496. Journal of the Acoustical Society of America, 85. Copyright 1989 American Institute of Physics)*

cross-sectional area are shown in Figure 6–4. As a result of individual differences in the dimensions of the ear canal, they cautioned against grouping data and obtaining a mean value, which would undoubtedly obscure some of the individual features that may be important while determining the sound pressure buildup within an ear canal. Contrary to the previous account of the ear canal dimensions as a straight tube, shown in Figure 6–2C (Hudde, 1983; Johansen, 1975), Stinson and Lawton (1989) pointed out that the ear canal is made up of a series of circular cylinders/slices of varying dimensions connected together to form the canal as shown in Figure 6–2A. Johansen (1975) and Stinson and Lawton (1989) undoubtedly provided a better understanding of the ear canal dimensions compared to previous studies. However, it would be impossible or extremely difficult to obtain ear canal impressions deep in living humans. To overcome this problem, Zemplenyi, Gilman, and Dirks (1985) developed a noninvasive optical method to measure the ear canal length. Their technique involved the use of a microscope. During the initial setting, the microscope was focused on the umbo of the eardrum as shown in Figure 6–5; the reading on the microscope arm was noted and then an

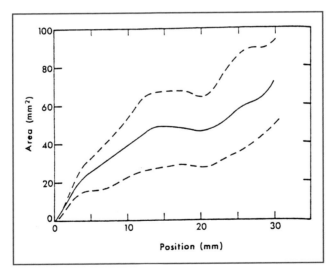

Figure 6–4. *Average cross-sectional area of the ear canal as a function of distance from the tympanic membrane. The solid line is the mean area and the dashed lines reflect the range of variations from the mean. (Reproduced with permission from Specification of the Geometry of the Human Ear Canal for the Prediction of Sound Pressure Level Distribution: M. R. Stinson and B. W. Lawton, 1989, p. 2500. Journal of the Acoustical Society of America, 85. Copyright 1989 American Institute of Physics)*

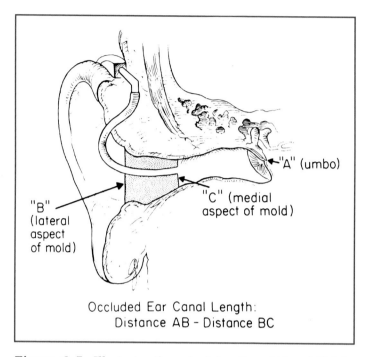

"A" (umbo)

"C" (medial aspect of mold)

"B" (lateral aspect of mold)

Occluded Ear Canal Length:
Distance AB – Distance BC

Figure 6–5. *Illustrates the actual locations "A" and "B" for the measurement of ear canal length. Length = "B-A." (Reproduced with permission from "Optical Method for the Measurement of Ear Canal Length" by J. Zemplenyi, S. Gilman, and D. Dirks,1985, pp. 2146–2147. Journal of the Acoustical Society of America, 78. Copyright 1985 American Institute of Physics)*

earmold was inserted into the ear canal. Following this, the microscope was refocused on the lateral aspect of the earmold (near the entrance of the ear canal). The microscope movement (i.e., the amount of shift in the position of the viewing arm from the first to the second measurement) indicated the length of the ear canal from the concha to the tympanic membrane at the umbo area. The optical method revealed an average canal length of 25 mm for males and 24 mm for females, a finding which is in agreement with previously published data (Johansen, 1975).

Radiologic Studies

Radiologic studies have also provided a noninvasive method to measure ear canal volume (Eckerdal, Ahlqvist, Alehagen, & Wing, 1978; Egolf, Nelson, Howell, & Larson, 1993; Qi, Liu, Lufty, Funnell, & Daniel, 2006; Van Willigan, 1976; Virapongse, Sarwar, Sasaki, & Kier, 1983). The studies by Egolf et al. (1993) and Qi et al. (2006) are noteworthy because of the innovative technique and differences in the ages. Egolf et al. (1993) procedure involved scanning the head of a cadaver sequentially at 1.0-mm intervals from the inferior to superior direction to obtain parallel transverse images (see Figure 6–6 for the actual procedure).

The second step involved cutting the transverse-images at 1.0-mm intervals starting at the tympanic membrane-ear canal junction and progressing laterally toward the concha to reconstruct the parasagittal images. The parasagittal images provided the cross-sectional dimension/ area of the ear canal; the cross-sectional dimensions at each 1.0 mm were then compared to cross-sectional areas of corresponding slices of an ear canal impression of the same ear. The actual values of the CAT images and the ear canal impression data and the differences between them are shown in Table 6–1. It appears that the cross-sectional values between

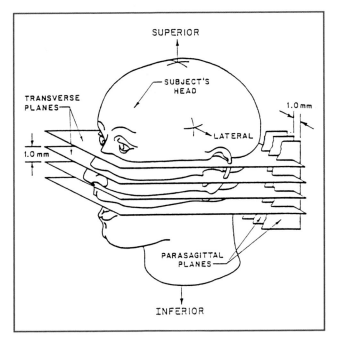

Figure 6–6. *Illustration of how the scanning was performed from inferior to superior direction to obtain transverse planes. The transverse data were cut to reveal parasagittal planes. Spacing between the planes is 1 mm. (Reproduced with permission from Quantifying Ear-canal Geometry with Multiple Computer-assisted Tomographic Scans: D. P. Egolf, D. K. Nelson, H. C. Howell, and V. D. Larson, 1993. p. 2810. Journal of the Acoustical Society of America, 93. Copyright 1993 American Institute of Physics)*

Table 6–1. Ear Canal Cross-Sectional Area Calculated from CT Scan Images and Ear Canal Impressions

Lateral Distance from Apex (in mm)	Cross-Section Area CT Images (in mm²)	Mold Imprints (in mm²)	Percent Difference (%)
1	—	—	NA
2	—	35.1	NA
3	—	27.1	NA
4	33.5	31.9	11.29
5	29.9	33.5	10.75
6	33.6	35.1	4.27
7	37.7	41.4	8.94
8	40.6	39.9	1.75
9	45.5	46.2	1.52
10	54.5	47.8	14.02
11	62.6	54.2	15.50
12	61.6	65.4	5.81
13	65.8	68.5	3.94
14	61.6	65.4	5.81
15	50.8	63.8	20.38
16	55.6	62.2	10.61
17	48.3	52.6	8.17
18	48.2	51.0	5.49
19	45.5	51.0	10.78
20	45.0	49.4	8.91
21	45.5	51.0	10.78
22	41.0	54.2	24.35
23	37.0	49.4	25.10
24	37.5	49.4	24.09
25	40.3	44.6	9.64
26	49.1	49.4	0.61
27	54.3	54.2	0.18
28	62.6	57.4	9.06
29	80.9	79.7	1.51
30	96.3	—	NA

Source: Data from Quantifying Ear-canal Geometry with Multiple Computer-assisted Tomographic Scans by D. P. Egolf, D. K. Nelson, H. C. Howell III, & V. D. Larson, 1993, p. 2818. *Journal of the Acoustical Society of America, 93,* 2809–2819.

the parasagittal images and the actual measurements were close and the differences ranged from 0.18% to 25.1% with a mean value of 9.65%. The volume estimates between CAT images (V_c) and mold impression (V_m) was also close; the difference was only 6.12%. They suggested that the CAT images provided measures closer to the actual volume of the ear canal than the immittance measure (see section immittance measures for details on the measurement techniques and the values) which had an error rate of >30.0% (Rabinowitz, 1977; Shanks & Lilly, 1981). Egolf et al. (1993) pointed out that the difference in the values between V_c and V_m may be due to the difficulty in differentiating the air/flesh interface in the CAT scanned images. The differences may also be due to shrinkage or expansion of the impression material used to make the earmolds. Regardless of these limitations and the expenses involved, it appears that their method still has several advantages over other methods. However, one concern of this procedure is that it exposed the subjects to radiation which can be harmful (Brenner & Hall, 2007); this might be overcome by the use of magnetic resonance imaging (MRI).

Qi et al. (2006) used a computer tomography (CT) scan to measure the geometry of the ear canal of a 22-day newborn. The objective of the measurement was to determine the ear canal volume changes as a function of differing atmospheric pressures. From the x-ray CT scan obtained they reconstructed the geometry model of the ear canal and tympanic membrane. The results from this study is comparable to previous findings in adults and newborns. Another observation from this study indicates that the ear canal wall and volume displacement are nonlinear with pressure changes from positive to negative 3 kPa. The measurements show that the canal dimensions are different compared to adults due to the elasticity of the skin lining the canal wall.

Acoustic Method

Ear canal geometry has also been calculated by measuring the sound pressure levels at different locations in the ear canal. Impetus to mathematical description of the ear canal comes from several investigations dealing with the functional area of vocal tracts (Attal, Chang, Mathews, & Tukey, 1978; Sondhi & Gopinath, 1971). Hudde (1983) described a method to determine the functional area of the ear canal by measuring sound pressure levels at more than two locations within the canal in human subjects. He considered the ear canal to be a conduit with varying cross section, and treated it as a lossless acoustic line. He assertained that exciting a duct by a sound source (i.e., a harmonic signal) would generate a pressure distribution described by the acoustic wave equation (Equation 1):

$$\frac{\partial^2 p}{\partial x^2} + \frac{1}{A(x)}\frac{dA(x)}{dx}\frac{\partial p}{\partial x} + \beta^2 p = 0.$$

Where, $p(x,\beta)$ is the acoustic pressure as a function of x, distance, β the angular wave number, and $v(x,\beta)$ the volume velocity. Here, $\beta = 2\pi f/c$, where f is the frequency, and c the velocity of sound.

From these values (i.e., the acoustic data) the next step is to determine the area of the ear canal ($A(x)$) by solving a linear system of equations and executing a simple iterative algorithm (Hudde, 1983, equation 2, p. 25) (Equation 2):

$$A(x) = A(0)\exp\left[-\int_0^x \left(\frac{\partial^2 p(\xi,\beta)}{\partial \xi^2} + \beta^2 p(\xi,\beta)\right)\bigg/ \frac{\partial p(\xi,\beta)}{\partial \xi}\, d\xi\right]$$

The key to determining the accurate area of the ear canal depends on measurements made at several locations in the ear canal. Hudde (1983) suggested that by presenting a broadband signal one can overcome the difficulties of making several measurements. The method he used for obtaining area included measuring sound pressure at three locations in the ear canal. The pressure measured at a given point is dependent on the frequency, the area function in the preceding stage, and the pressure level at the previous location. From the three measurements he obtained the area of the ear canal (Equation 3):

$$A_N = \left(1 + \sum_{j=1}^{Z_1(N)} z_j\right)\bigg/ \sum_{j=1}^{Z_2(N)} x_j$$

$$Z_{j,n} = \sum_{j=1}^{i} z_{j,n+1} - A_{n+1}\sum_{j=1}^{f} x_{j,n+1} + 1$$

$$x_{j,n} = \sum_{j=1}^{i} x_{j,n+1} - A_{n+1}^{-1}\left(1 + \sum_{j=1}^{i-1} z_{j,n+1}\right)$$

$$A_n = \left(1 + \sum_{j=1}^{Z_1(n)} z_{j,n}\right)\bigg/ \sum_{j=1}^{Z_2(n)} x_{j,n}$$

The main advantage of this method is that the formula is linear and the computations are simple, and provide a good approximation of the actual area of the ear canal. In spite of their good approximation of the area functions, he cautioned that area functions should be measured using broader bandwidth signals for greater accuracy. However, even though Hudde (1983) recognized that the ear canal is a nonhomogeneous tube, he did not recognize the importance of the curvature of the canal while calculating the geometry.

The work of Hudde (1983) provided the beginnings of determining area function using sound pressure developed with the canal. An ear canal is an irregular tube; it varies in dimension and direction (S-shaped). Therefore, sound traveling in such a tube will have a different amount of reflection due to irregularities. Hence the sound transmission within the canal is a total sum of sound pressure developed by reflected and propagated sounds at any given frequency. It is beyond the scope of this book to describe various equations used to measure the pressure development in the canal; an interested reader can review the excellent articles listed in the references section (Hudde & Schmidt, 2009; Stinson & Daigle, 2005).

A less complicated method to determine the length of the canal was proposed by Chan and Giesler (1990). Their technique involved measuring sound pressure levels at various locations within the ear canal due to a broadband signal and determining the maxima and minima at different frequencies. It is known that at any one frequency, the pressure amplitude reaches the minima at a distance of one-quarter the wavelength of the signal from the tympanic membrane (i.e., standing waves). These pressure minima appear as notches in the spectrum from the pressure measurements conducted at different locations. The quarter-wavelength corresponding to this frequency can be used to estimate the distance from the tympanic membrane. The distance can be estimated by the following formula (Equation 4):

$$l = c/4f$$

where l = estimated distance, c = speed of sound in air, and f = the notch frequency.

The notch frequency was determined by subtracting the recording at one location from that of the next; doing so will eliminate the similarities and enhance the differences. The notches and peaks can be used to determine the length of ear canal. The canal length as measured from the acoustic method was compared to the actual measurements obtained from the optical method described by Zemplenyi et al. (1985), and the acoustic method fell within ±2 mm of the optical method. This suggests that the acoustic method is as reliable as the optical method to measure the ear canal length.

Immittance Measurements

With the advent of commercially available electroacoustic immittance devices, the ear canal volume is measured as part of routine clinical immittance testing. The actual volume measured in this case is the column of air between the probe tip and tympanic membrane; therefore, one should not mistake the total ear canal volume obtained by other procedures to be the same as that of immittance measures. The tympanometric estimate of the ear canal volume is performed to calculate the impedance of the air column between the probe tip and the tympanic membrane. Then the impedance of the air column is subtracted from the total impedance to determine the immittance at the tympanic membrane. The theoretical underpinnings of immittance measurement suggest that when the tympanic membrane is made stiffer by altering the pressure (+400 da Pa to −400 da Pa), the impedance of the eardrum and the middle ear system goes to infinity (for practical purposes it is considered to be infinite), thus enabling the measurement of the ear canal volume. Controversy exists regarding the use of tympanometric procedures to estimate ear canal volume. Researchers have suggested that when the ear canal is subjected to pressure variations the shape changes; ear canal pressures as high/low as ±400 da Pa are not enough to drive the middle ear impedance to infinity to decouple the outer ear from the middle ear system.

However, several studies have attempted to determine the relationship between the tympanometric estimate of ear canal volume to the physical volume of the ear canal obtained between the probe tip and the tympanic membrane. Rabinowitz (1977) estimated the ear canal volume at ±400 da Pa for a 220-Hz probe tone, and suggested that the tympanometric volume estimate (0.76 mL) was 33% higher than the actual volume (0.57 mL). Shanks and Lilly (1981) also evaluated the ear canal volume using tympanometric procedures. The ear canal volume from susceptance tympanograms recorded for two probe frequencies (220 and 660 Hz) and several pressure gradients (between ±400 da Pa) was compared to the actual ear canal volume measured by filling alcohol into the free space between the probe tip and the tympanic membrane. They reported that the tympanometric procedures overestimated the actual physical volume; the largest difference was noted for 220 Hz at 200 da Pa (39.0%), and the smallest error was reported at −400 da Pa for both

220 and 660 Hz. In general, the 660-Hz probe tone more closely reflected the actual volume (10% error) than the 220-Hz tone (24% error). The reason for the differences in the volume estimate between 220 and 660-Hz probe frequencies was attributed to the variation in the reactance of the middle ear system at these two frequencies. Shanks and Lilly (1981) suggested that "as the probe frequency approaches closer to the middle ear resonance (800–1200 Hz), the reactance values recorded in the plane of the probe are contaminated less by middle ear effects, and thus provide a more accurate estimate of ear canal volume" (Shanks & Lilly, 1981, p. 562). Therefore, if one is interested in measuring the ear canal volume, it is advisable to use probe frequencies closer to the middle ear resonant frequency in order to reduce the variability between the physical volume and the measured volume.

Recently, Rasetshwane and Neely (2011) proposed a method to determine the area function of the ear canal by acoustic impedance at the entrance of the ear canal. The method is based on a solution to the inverse problem in which measurements of impedance are used to calculate reflectance, which is then used to determine the area function of the canal. They recruited 24 subjects with normal hearing and middle ear functions; however, only the data from 21 subjects were used for data analysis. A custom-built impedance measuring device was used and the stimulus was a wideband linear-swept frequency chirp signal. From the load impedance data, reflectance was measured by Equation 5:

$$R\,(x,\,\omega) = \frac{Z_L\,(x,\,\omega) - Z_0\,(x)}{Z_L\,(x,\,\omega) + Z_0\,(x)}$$

Where Z_0 is the characteristic impedance of the ear canal. The frequency-domain reflectance was calculated from the measured load impedance using Equation 5. It is a known fact that from frequency domain reflectance one can extract the time domain reflectance by applying the inverse Fourier transform. The time domain reflectance is important, since it shows the magnitude of the sound pulse as it travels from the entrance of the ear canal to the eardrum, and the reflected sound pulse from the eardrum as it travels back to the entrance of the ear canal.

Theoretically, this procedure is equivalent to the process of introducing a short duration sound pulse into the ear canal, and measuring its response as a function of time. This time reflectance information gives direct information about the ear canal area because it shows the reflectance of each part of the ear canal as sound pulse travels along it. From the reflectance of the incident pulse of each part of the ear canal the change of the canal area can be calculated (Rasteswane & Neely, 2011).

Although a lot of conceptual concerns regarding this process exist, the important one is refining the calculations and next concerns the texture of the canal. However, the findings of the average ear canal area function from their study correspond to the previous findings of Johasen (1975), Stinson and Lawton (1989), and Egolf et al. (1993). They claim that the ear canal area function obtained from reflectance is accurate, fast, noninvasive, and reproducible. They caution that inadequate spatial resolution and excessive sensitivity to analysis parameter might limit the accuracy of the method.

In response to the question of, how does one measures ear canal geometry, the explanation provided so far clearly suggests that there are several techniques to do so. These methods have undergone considerable changes and the newer techniques are in the process of further refinement. Each description of the ear canal reflects an increase in the accuracy of measurement over its predecessor. In quantifying the dimensions of the ear canal, particularly the volume, the sophistication has increased from considering the ear canal as just a simple cavity to a cylindrical tube to a serial connection of circular cylinders, each representing one thin cross sectional slice of the ear canal. The historic progression of ear canal models can be described as: (1) a simple cavity, (2) a circular cylinder, and finally (3) a serial connection of circular cylinders. The published findings on ear canal geometry from several investigators are presented in Table 6–2.

Contributions of Pinna and Ear Canal to Sound Pressure Transformation from Free-Field to the Tympanic Membrane

According to Shaw (1975), the factors that govern the sound transformation from free-field to the tympanic membrane were divided into two major areas: (1) the head, torso, and pinna flange acting as diffracting bodies; and (2) the concha and the ear canal acting as resonators. Stated differently, when the outer ear is excited by a broadband signal (e.g., broadband noise) from the free-field, certain frequencies are emphasized and others are not. The magnitude difference in the amount of sound pressure at the tympanic membrane to that of the free-field is due to the pressure gain achieved by the outer ear (i.e., the pinna and ear canal). Since the focus of this chapter is the pressure gain attained by the ear canal, a majority of the discussion will be directed toward the acoustic properties of the ear canal; however, contributions from pinna, especially the concha, will be included when necessary.

Table 6–2. Summary of the Ear Canal Geometry from Several Published Reports

Investigators	Parameters and Type of Measurement	Dimensions	
Johnson (1975)	Length of the ear canal Physical measurement	25.7 mm (±1.9 mm)	
Djuspland and Zwislocki (1972)	Length of the ear canal Physical measurement	Male	23.8 mm
		Female	22.0 mm
		Combined	23.0 mm
Zemplenyi et al. (1985)	Length of the ear canal Optical method	Male	25.0 mm
		Female	24.0 mm
Chan and Giesler (1990)	Length of the ear canal Optical method	Male	23.4 (±2.1) mm
		Female	19.7 (±0.9) mm
	Acoustic method	Male	23.4 (±1.9) mm
		Female	20.9 (±0.9) mm
Salvinelli et al. (1991)	Length of the ear canal	Male	25.2 (±2.6) mm
		Female	22.4 (±2.3) mm
		Total	23.5 (±2.5) mm
Salvinelli et al. (1991)	Longest diameter	Male	9.7 (±1.5) mm
		Female	8.5 (±0.7) mm
		Total	9.4 (±1.5) mm
Salvinelli et al. (1991)	Shortest diameter	Male	5.1 (±0.7) mm
		Female	4.4 (±0.3) mm
		Total	4.8 (±0.5) mm
Johnson (1975)	Ear canal volume	1,014.0 ± 15.4 mm^3	
Egolf et al. (1993)	Ear canal volume	CAT volume	1211.51 mm^3
		Mold volume	1290.49 mm^3
Smelt et al. (1988)	Tympanic membrane Longest diameter	Male	9.8 mm
		Female	9.5 mm
		Total	9.6
Smelt et al. (1988)	Shortest diameter	Male	8.5 mm
		Female	8.9 mm
		Total	8.6 mm

continues

Table 6–2. continued

Investigators	Parameters and Type of Measurement	Dimensions	
Salvinelli et al. (1991)	Tympanic membrane Longest diameter	Male	9.7 mm (±1.8 mm)
		Female	9.2 mm (±1.2 mm)
		Total	9.4 mm (±1.5 mm)
Salvinelli et al. (1991)	Shortest diameter	Male	8.9 mm (±1.0 mm)
		Female	8.4 mm (±0.7 mm)
		Total	8.6 mm (±0.9 mm)
Smelt et al. (1988)	Tympanic membrane Antero-inferior angle	Male	17°
		Female	17°
		Total	17°
Salvinelli et al. (1991)		Male	18° ±2°
		Female	20° ±2°
		Total	19° ±2°
Smelt et al. (1988)	Tympanic membrane central canal axis angle	Male	44°
		Female	48°
		Total	47°
Salvinelli et al. (1991)	Tympanic membrane central canal axis angle	Male	42° ±3°
		Female	45° ±4°
		Total	43.4° ±4°
Qi et al. (2006)	Roof length (Newborn)	16 mm	
	Floor length (Newborn)	22.5 mm	
	Canal diameter (Newborn)	1.6–4.8 mm	
Rasetshwane & Neely (2011)	Canal length	14.28–29.36 mm (mean length 24.08 mm)	
	Volume of the canal	372–1464 mm^3 (mean volume 843 mm^3)	

An ear canal is a tube that is opened at one end (concha region) and closed at the other (tympanic membrane). It contains air and the body of air will resonate in response to sounds of various frequencies. The frequency that matches the natural resonant frequency of the ear canal is amplified compared to other frequencies. The wavelength of the fundamental resonance of the ear canal is 4 times its length. That means only one-quarter of the wave can fit into the tube at any one pass; thus, the ear canal is called a quarter-wave resonator. The wavelengths for various frequencies are listed in Table 6–3, which shows that the lower the frequency, the longer the wavelength and vice versa. This suggests that for lower frequencies, one-quarter wavelength is longer than the length of the ear canal (25 mm) and the opposite is true for higher frequencies.

The resonant frequency of the ear canal can be calculated mathematically by the following formula (Equation 6):

$$f = c/4l$$

in which f = resonant frequency of the ear canal, c = velocity of sound in air (34,400 cm), and l = length of the ear canal (25 mm). Given the values of the velocity of the sound in air and the length of the ear canal,

Table 6–3. Computed Wave Lengths at Octave and Interoctave Frequencies from 0.1 to 10.0 kHz

Frequency Hz	Wavelength $y = c/f*$	Wavelength "y" in centimeters
100 Hz	34,400/100	344 cm
200 Hz	34,400/200	172 cm
400 Hz	34,400/400	86 cm
500 Hz	34,400/500	68.8 cm
1000 Hz	34,400/1,000	34.4 cm
2000 Hz	34,400/2,000	17.2 cm
4000 Hz	34,400/4,000	8.6 cm
6000 Hz	34,400/6,000	5.7 cm
8000 Hz	34,400/8,000	4.3 cm
10000 Hz	34,400/10,000	3.44 cm
12000 Hz	34,400/12,000	2.86 cm
14000 Hz	34,400/14,000	2.45 cm
16000 Hz	34,400/16,000	2.15 cm
18000 Hz	34,400/18,000	1.91 cm
20000 Hz	34,400/20,000	1.72 cm

*where c = speed of sound in air (cm), and f = frequency

one can determine the resonant frequency of the ear canal as follows: f = 34,400/(4 × 2.5); f = 34,400/100; f = 3440 Hz (resonant frequency of the ear canal). Therefore, the resonant frequency of an ear canal 25 mm in length is 3440 Hz. It is important to remember that any variation in the length of the canal can alter the resonant frequency. Consequently, the exact dimensions of the canal, especially the length, should be specified before calculating the resonant frequency of a given ear canal.

The literature is replete with excellent articles on acoustic properties of the ear canal based on measurements made inside the human ear canal, as well as data from mathematical and physical models (Djupesland & Zwislocki, 1972; Farmer-Fedor & Rabbitt, 2002; Gilman & Dirks, 1986; Hammershoi & Moller, 1196; Hellstorm & Axelson, 1993; Hudde & Schmidt, 2009; Khanna & Stinson, 1985; Mehrgardt & Mellert, 1977; Middlebrooks, 1989a, 1989b; Rabbitt & Friedrich, 1991; Rabbitt & Holmes, 1989; Shaw, 1966, 1969, 1974a, 1975, 1980; Shaw & Teranishi, 1968; Shaw & Villancourt, 1985; Stinson, 1985; Stinson & Daigle, 2005, 2007; Stinson & Khanna, 1994; Stinson, Shaw, & Lawton, 1982; Teranishi & Shaw, 1968; Wiener & Ross, 1946). The most common measurement of the ear canal function has been the magnitude of pressure difference (P_T/P_{SF}) between the sound pressure at the tympanic membrane (P_T) compared to that in sound-field (P_{SF}). As mentioned before, the largest pressure gain occurs usually at the resonant frequency of the ear canal.

Wiener and Ross (1946), in their classic study, placed a probe-tube microphone at two locations in the ear canal, one near the tympanic membrane and the other halfway between the tympanic membrane and the concha. At these two locations, they measured sound pressure distribution within the ear canal from a free-field sound presented at three angles of incidence: 0, 45, and 90 degrees in the horizontal plane. The difference in the pressure between free-field locations and that of the microphones placements revealed variables gains at different frequencies. The most obvious pressure gain across a range of frequencies was 10 to 15 between 2.0 to 4.0 kHz. with a maximum increment of 17 to 22 dB at 3.0 kHz. The important findings of this study are: (1) the outer ear (i.e., concha and ear canal) acts as a resonator and the amount of resonance provided is up to 20 dB between frequencies 2.0 to 5.0 kHz, and (2) the sound source has a differential effect on the amount of pressure developed within the canal across frequencies.

Subsequently, Shaw (1974a, 1974b), in a series of experiments, appraised our understanding of ear canal acoustics and supplemented data on the interaction of frequency and several azimuthal positions on the average sound pressure transformation from free-field to the tympanic membrane. The family of curves shown in Figure 6–7 is based on

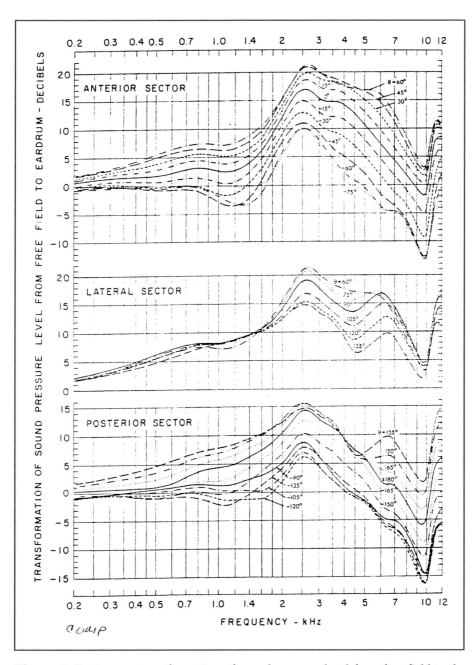

Figure 6–7. *Average transformation of sound pressure level from free-field to the ear canal across different frequencies as a function of azimuths presented from frontal, lateral, and posterior sectors. (Reproduced with permission from "Transformation of Sound Pressure Level from Free Field to the Eardrum in the Horizontal Plane" by E. A. G Shaw, 1974b, p. 1865. Journal of the Acoustical Society of America, 56. Copyright 1974 American Institute of Physics)*

several measurements at different laboratories around the world; it is obvious from the data that the primary ear canal resonance is at 2.6 kHz. Again, it is noticeable that the differences in the amount of sound pressure within the ear canal compared to the free-field SPL were dependent on the angle of incidence (e.g., sound pressure difference at 2.6 kHz was as much as 21 dB at 45° to 60° azimuth compared to 17 dB for a sound at 0° frontal plane).

The relationship between the structural components of the outer ear to the pressure gain has been addressed by Shaw and his colleagues (1974b; Shaw & Teranishi, 1968; Teranishi & Shaw, 1968). To fully appreciate the contributions of each components of the outer ear, Teranishi and Shaw (1968) developed a physical model of simple cylindrical cavities to reflect the resonances of concha, pinna flange, ear canal, and, additionally, acoustic damping was added to simulate the effects of the tympanic membrane. The response curves at four stages of development are shown in Figures 6–8A through 6–8D). Figure 6–8A represents the resonance of concha; the family of curves shown reflects the response of the cavity to sounds originating from different directions, normal incidence (solid line), 45° in front (dotted line), behind (long dashes), above (dot-dash), and below (short dash). The curves in sections B, C, and D illustrate the effects of adding the pinna flange, ear canal, and the tympanic membrane to the first cavity (i.e., the concha). As these components were added, the resonance peaks systematically shifted from higher to lower frequencies. The most salient effect in the resonance peaks can be noted when the ear canal was added to the replica. The largest peak is observed at 3.0 kHz, which fits the resonance frequency value obtained from mathematical computations discussed earlier.

Based on measurements made in the replicas and occluded ear canals in humans, Shaw (1974a) estimated the effect of various structures on the pressure gain. He suggested that the total pressure "T" shown in Figure 6–9 is the resultant sum of contributions of several structures which includes the torso, the neck, the head, the pinna flange, the concha, and the ear canal. Contributions of each structure are based on the interaction of size of the structure and the wave length (λ). Therefore, for frequencies below 1.0 kHz the gain in sound pressure is only 5 dB, mostly due to the contributions of torso, neck, and head. At frequencies between 1.0 kHz and 3.0 kHz, the ear canal is the single most contributor, and above 3.0 kHz small structures such as the concha begin to play a major role in the pressure gain. Thus, the sound reaching the tympanic membrane reflects the cumulative effect of the pressure gain attained by individual components, and it is reported to be arounnd15 to 20 dB between 1.5 to 7.0 kHz (see T curve in Figure 6–9).

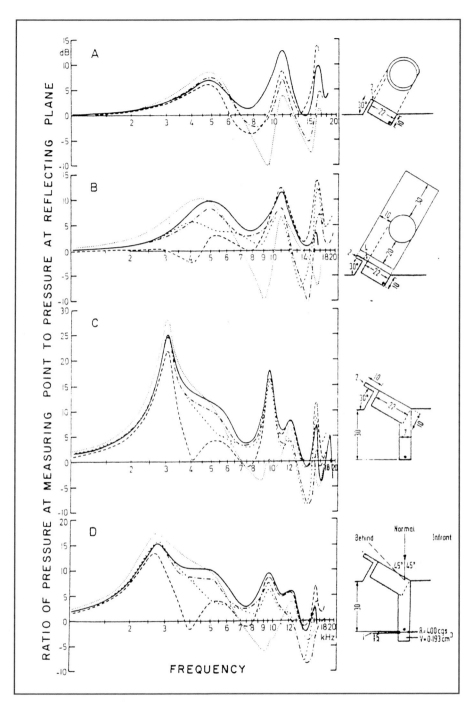

Figure 6–8. *Response from a replica of human outer ear and tympanic membrane. The curves in each figure reflect the location of the sound source, normal incidence (solid line), source at 45° azimuth (dotted line), behind (long dash), above (dot-dash), and below (short dash). **A.** Response properties of the concha. **B.** Concha and pinna flange added. **C.** Ear canal added to A, B, and D. The combined effects of A, B, and C, and the tympanic membrane. (Reproduced with permission from "External-Ear Acoustic Models with Simple Geometry"by R. Terinishi and E. A. G. Shaw, 1968, p. 258. Copyright 1968 American Institute of Physics)*

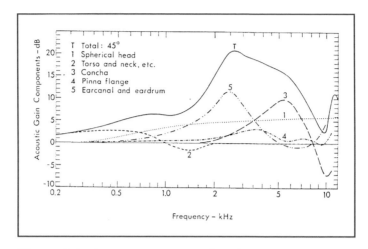

Figure 6–9. *Average pressure gain from human torso, neck, and outer ear to sound presented at 45° azimuth (Reproduced with permission from "The External Ear" by E. A. G. Shaw, 1974a, p. 468. In W. D. Keidel and W. Neff (Eds.),* Handbook of Sensory Physiology *(Vol. 1). Copyright 1974 Springer-Verlag)*

Answers to the question how much does the pinna and ear canal contribute to the pressure transformation from the free-field to the tympanic membrane can be summarized as follows:

1. The combined resonance of the pinna and ear canal provides a gain of 20–30 dB between 1.5 to 7.0 kHz.

2. The major components responsible for the resonance of the outer ear are the concha and the ear canal.

3. The magnitude of sound pressure within the canal is directional dependent. A sound originating from 45° azimuth appears to produce the largest pressure gain at the resonance frequency compared to sound from other locations.

Factors That Can Alter the Sound Pressure Transformation from Free-Field to the Tympanic Membrane

It has been shown that several factors can affect the pressure gain achieved by the ear canal. Among them the most important factors are: (1) differences in ear canal dimensions due to developmental changes;

(2) location of the sound source; (3) cerumen accumulation, the presence of a foreign body, and integrity of the tympanic membrane; and (4) location of the recording microphone in the ear canal. Location is an important procedural consideration because the position will influence the absolute level of the recorded sound pressure in the ear canal, especially for high frequencies. Additional factors, such as the impedance at the plane of the tympanic membrane and ear canal, have been attributed to altering the sound pressure level within the canal.

Differences in Ear Canal Size

There are substantial differences between adults and infants regarding head size, pinna size, and ear canal dimensions. Developmental studies have indicated that the shape and size of the ear canal change from the postnatal period to 7–9 years of age (see Chapter 2). Nevertheless, infants and children are being fitted with hearing aids at an early age based on electroacoustic measurements made on KEMAR or the typical adult head. Perhaps this is because there are considerably fewer studies on the sound pressure measurements within the ear canals of young children and infants compared to adults.

Despite the difficulties associated with recording sound pressure inside the ear canal of children and infants, few studies have demonstrated changes in ear canal resonance as a function of age (Bentler, 1989; Dempster & McKenzie, 1990; Kruger, 1987; Keef, Bulen, Campbell, & Burns, 1994). Noteworthy is the work of Kruger (1987), who measured the diffuse-field to ear canal transfer function in 26 children from birth to 37 months of age. She reported that the ear canal resonance was significantly higher in newborns; it ranged between 5.3 to 7.2 kHz and decreased to the adult value of 2.7 kHz by the second year of life as shown in Figure 6–10. In addition, Kruger (1987) calculated the "effective length" from the resonance frequency measurements to imply that the ear canal in infants is shorter than that of adults; the differences noted were as much as 3 times (10 mm in children to 32 mm in adults). However, caution must be exercised when comparing the "effective length" and the actual physical length, because the "effective length" tends to be longer than the physical length by a factor of 25%.

Additional data about the ear canal resonance characteristics of children aged 3 to 13 years were provided by Bentler (1989). The average ear canal resonance characteristics for children as a function of frequency were found to be similar to that of the adults except for a small difference of 3–5 dB above 3.0 kHz. She suggested that the higher values for the

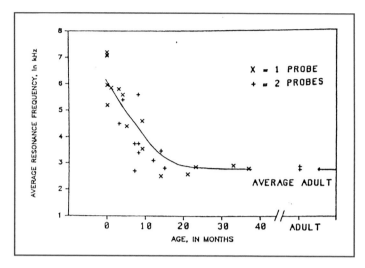

Figure 6–10. *Resonance frequency plotted as a function of age. (Reproduced with permission from "An Update on the External Ear Resonance in Infants and Young Children" by B. Kruger, 1987, p. 334.* Ear and Hearing, 8. *Copyright 1987 Williams & Wilkins)*

children might be due to the difference in the shape of the ear canal and pinna in children. The results of her findings were compared to Shaw's (1974b) data for adult subjects and she concluded that the adult model can be applied to children above 3 years of age. Dempster and Mackenzie (1990) measured ear canal resonance in 250 children aged 3–12 years, and reported an ear canal resonance near 3.0 kHz for children below the age of 4 years, and the adult values were achieved by the age of 7 years. This finding is significantly different from the earlier observations of Kruger (1987) and Bentler (1989) where the adult values were recorded by the age of 3 years. A criticism raised by Bentler (1991) about Dempster and Mackenzie's (1990) data was that the comparisons were made between age and resonance frequency without due consideration to either the ear canal volume or the length. It is possible that variations in ear canal size, rather than age, might have contributed to the differences in the resonant frequency as considerable intersubject variations are noted in ear canal geometry within the range group.

In another study, Keefe et al. (1994) measured the ear canal transfer function in a diffuse sound field for human infants aged 1, 6, 12, and 24 months. They noted two peaks in the 2.0 to 6.0 kHz range reflecting the combined resonance of the ear canal and concha. The ear canal resonance decreased from 4.4 kHz at 1 month to 2.9 kHz at 24 months; correspondingly, the concha resonance also decreased from 5.5 kHz at 1 month to

4.5 kHz at 24 months. They proposed a simple two-cylinder model to predict the sound transformation function in children. The above findings suggest that the ear canal resonance decreases form the postnatal stage to 2 years of life. The main variable responsible for the decrease in resonant frequency appears to be the volume of the ear canal.

In summary, it is important to realize these individual differences within infant, children, and adult groups, as well as across groups when determining electroacoustic characteristics for selecting and fitting hearing aids.

Location of the Sound Source

The location of the sound source can vary either in horizontal (interaural) or vertical (above or below) directions, and a combination of these two directions can produce spatial patterns where the sound may originate from several locations in the auditory space. Studies have shown that the ear canal pressure gain is directional: the gain varies with the source (Hellstrom & Axelson, 1993; Middlebrooks, 1999a, 1999b; Middlebrooks, Makous, & Green, 1989; Musicant, Chan, & Hind, 1990; Shaw, 1974a). Most of the earlier studies in humans investigated the directional pressure sensitivity within the ear canal in the horizontal plane (Shaw, 1974a, 1974b; Wiener & Ross, 1946). However, some of the recent measurements of pressure gain demonstrate a large dependence on vertical as well as the azimuth on ear's response to tones of different frequencies (Hellstrom & Axelson, 1993; Middlebrooks, 1999a, 1999b); Middlebrooks et al., 1989, in humans; Musicant et al., 1990, in cats). A quantitative measurement of the direction-dependent pressure differences within the ear canal was examined by Hellstrom and Alexson (1993). They measured the transfer function (microphone placed at 1–3 mm from the tympanic membrane) from free-field to the tympanic membrane in 19 subjects for sounds (a 1/3 octave band filtered noise from 0.2 to 20.0 kHz) presented through speakers located at 24 horizontal (azimuths 0° to 315°) and 3 vertical (+45° E, 00° E, –45° E) positions (total 72 positions). The averaged results across subjects from 8 azimuthal (azimuths 0° to 315° in 45°) and 3 vertical (+45° E, 00° E, –45° E) locations are illustrated in Figure 6–11. The ordinate in Figure 6–11 is the pressure gain within the ear canal compared to sound field and the abscissa refers to the frequency of the stimuli (0.2 to 20 kHz). The most prominent finding from these curves (see Figure 6–11) is that the direction related differences in the sound pressure gain occur at frequencies above the resonant frequency of the ear canal.

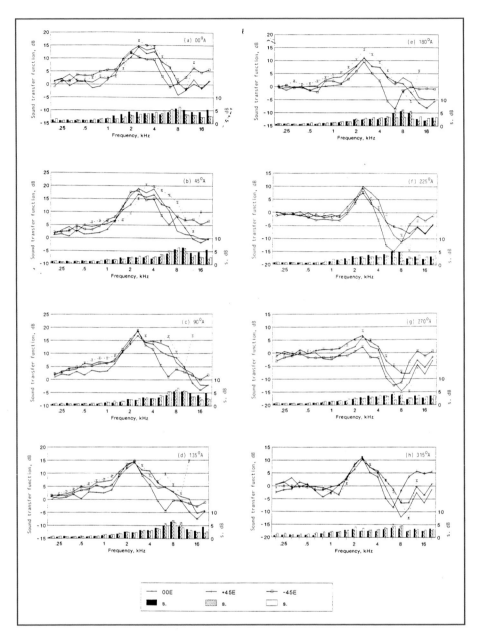

Figure 6–11. *Sound pressure transfer function from free-field to tympanic membrane. Plots A–H sound pressure levels measured by a microphone placed near tympanic membrane to sound presented from 8 horizontal (0–315° A) and 3 vertical (0 ±45° E). The dotted line shown in the plots are taken from Shaw and Villancourt (1985). (Reproduced with permission from "Miniature Microphone Probe Tube Measurements in the External Auditory Canal" by P. A. Hellstrom and A. Axelson, 1993, p. 915.* Journal of the Acoustical Society of America. *Copyright 1993 American Institute of Physics)*

These findings are in agreement with earlier studies of Shaw & Villancourt (1985) (see dotted line in Figure 6–11). They reported that direction dependent pressure differences was greater than 20 dB across subjects at certain frequencies (between 6.3 and 10 kHz) and the variations can be as much as 30 dB in the same subject for sounds arriving from different locations. These intersubject pressure differences may suggest that the variations might be due to differences in the dimensions of ear canal and pinna; however, there are no studies on such interactions to report at this time.

In summary, the pinna and ear canal transforms the free-field sound pressure augmenting the directionality associated with it by adding considerable pressure gain at different higher frequencies. These properties are ultimately important for the spatial perception of sound. From several studies (Hellstrom & Axelson, 1993; Middlebrooks et.al., 1989; Middlebrooks, 1992; Shaw, 1974a, 1974b;) it is now clearly established that the monaural localization of sound is linked to the direction-dependent filtering of sound by the external ear which occurs at frequencies above 4.0 kHz.

Effects of Cerumen, Foreign Bodies, and Tympanic Membrane Perforations

An occluded ear canal (either partial of complete) is assumed to change the volume of the ear canal. It is a common finding in audiology clinics that patients' ear canals are impacted or occluded with cerumen. The degree to which these impactions cause alterations in the resonance properties of the ear canal is still an unanswered question. The only study to date that has looked at the effects of ear canal occlusion is by Chandler (1964) who measured the relationship between the amount of blockage to the amount of threshold shift across audiometric frequencies (see Figure 4–1). Based on his findings, he concluded that ear canal blockage resulted in threshold shift; a complete occlusion produced an average threshold shift of 30 dB at frequencies above 2.0 kHz. It is apparent that the differences in thresholds across frequencies are due to loss of resonance of the ear canal.

Tympanic membrane (TM) perforations can also have rather dramatic effects on the resonant frequencies of the ear canal. Moryl, Danhauer, and Di Bartolomeo (1992) found that the size and shape of the ear canal resonant peaks varied considerably depending upon the size of TM perforation. While smaller TM perforations produced more similar resonant peaks to those of nonperforated TMs, ears having large

TM perforation exhibited bimodal peaks separated by large troughs that were often above or below the normally expected range of 2.7 kHz. They also showed that resonant peaks in ears with large TM perforations became more normal looking after surgical closure of the perforation. They suggested that their findings could have important implications for selecting and fitting hearing aids to ears with perforation.

Thus, audiologists and others involved in auditory function measurements must also pay attention to changes in ear canal volume due to the presence of cerumen, foreign objects, or tympanic membrane perforations.

Location of the Probe Tube Within the Canal

An important procedural consideration while measuring the sound pressure in the ear canal is the placement of the probe tube/microphone within the canal. The magnitude of the sound pressure measured inside the ear canal is highly dependent on the exact location of the point of measurement, due to the presence of standing waves and the variations in the shape of the canal. Consequently, location-dependent variations can produce substantial differences in the sound pressure recorded inside the ear canal, especially for frequencies greater than 3.0 kHz.

The reasons for pressure variations or the presence of standing waves within the ear canal is detailed as follows. When a sound impinges on the tympanic membrane some of the energy is dissipated, some is reflected back, and most of the energy is transmitted through the tympanic membrane (TM) into the middle ear. The reflection of energy is due to impedance differences between the tympanic membrane (Z-tympanic membrane) and the transmission line (Z-ear canal). The interaction between the reflected and incident waves results in standing waves with pressure maxima and minima at different points along the ear canal (Dirks & Kincaid, 1987; Gilman & Dirks, 1986; Lawton & Stinson, 1986; Stinson & Khanna, 1994; Stinson & Shaw, 1985). A schematic representation of the standing wave patterns in a rigid-walled cylindrical tube is shown in Figure 6–12 (Gilman & Dirks, 1986). Plotted on the abscissa is the location of the probe microphone with respect to tympanic membrane, while the ordinate shows the difference in sound pressure measured, (i.e., the amount of sound pressure underestimated by the probe microphone to the level present at the tympanic membrane). These pressure minima and maxima are at different locations along the

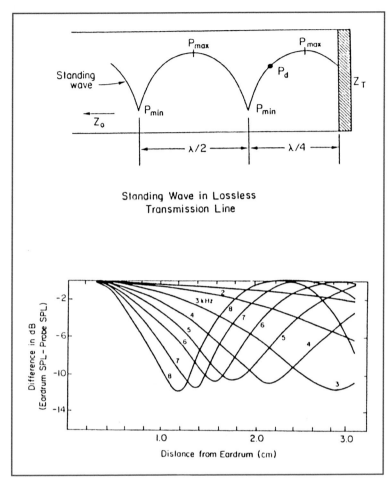

Figure 6–12. Top panel: *Illustrates a standing wave in a lossless tube. Z₀ and Z_T are impedances of the tube (line) and tympanic membrane. The P min and max are pressure minima and maxima for a soundwave of length (l). Note the first Pmin is observed at 1/4l. (Reproduced with permission from "Basic Acoustic Considerations of Ear Canal Probe Measurements" by D. Dirks and G. Kincaid, 1987, p. 61S, Ear and Hearing, 8[Suppl. 5]. Copyright 1987 Williams and Wilkins).* Bottom panel: *Family of standing waves for frequencies 1.0 to 8.0 kHz. The negative dB values refer to the difference between the eardrum- and probe-measured sound pressure levels (P min) at different locations along the ear canal from the tympanic membrane. Note the shift in Pmin toward the eardrum at higher frequencies. (Reproduced with permission from "Acoustics of Ear-canal Measurement of Eardrum SPL in simulators" by S. Gilman and D. Dirks, 9186, p. 786.* Journal of the Acoustical Society of America, 80. *Copyright 1986 American Institute of Physics)*

length of the canal dependent on frequency; the first minima is usually observed at a distance equal to the quarter-wavelength (l/4) of the frequency of the stimulus. For example, a probe microphone placed at 1.0 cm away from the tympanic membrane can change the sound press values by as much as about 10 dB for a 8.0 kHz tone compared to a placement closer to the TM. For frequencies below 3.0 kHz the pressure maxima or minima is negligible or insignificant because the minima of the standing waves falls outside the length of the ear canal; however, at higher frequencies, the number of pressure minima and maxima increase monotonically with the frequency.

In addition to the location of the microphone, the impedance of the tympanic membrane and the middle ear has significant effects on the specific location of the pressure maxima and minima within the ear canal. Gilman and Dirks (1986) reported that high and low impedance systems tend to produce minima at different locations compared to the normal system. The high impedance systems appears to produce minima closer to the tympanic membrane, whereas low impedance systems produce minima at locations farther from the tympanic membrane.

In clinical practice, the probe microphone should be placed closer to the tympanic membrane; a distance of 5 mm from the tympanic membrane can achieve the needed accuracy of measurement even for high frequencies. When performing repeated measurements the probe/ microphone must be placed at the same location. Additionally, any middle ear problems should be noted during the ear canal measurements; if possible, the results should be repeated after any abnormal middle ear conditions have been resolved.

Currently Available Outer Ear Simulator/Couplers for Acoustic Measurements

Artificial ears, or couplers, as they are known in the literature, have been used in audiology and acoustic research for several reasons, most often to calibrate earphones (either circumaural or insert) to measure hearing aid output, and to perform acoustic measurements during psychoacoustic or physiologic experiments. The use of acoustic couplers/artificial ear over real ear has traditionally been due to the desire to provide standardized measurements and to overcome limitations in performing tests on humans (either due to patient discomfort or restrictions on using human subjects for some tests). Early on, it became necessary for researchers to develop a physical system that was capable of simulating the human outer ear and tympanic membrane. Although the terms "artificial ear" and "couplers" have been used interchangeably in the literature, it is important to know the differences between them. According to Bruel et al. (1975) coupler is a device which connects the earphone to a microphone. For the coupler or a device to be called an artificial ear, it should offer the same load as that of a real ear. That means the sound pressure developed in a coupler/device should match the pressure developed in the real ear in amplitude and frequency. Thus, the available devices for calibration and acoustic measurements can be grouped into four categories: (1) the coupler, (2) the artificial ear, (3) the earlike coupler, and (4) the Manikin also known as the KEMAR.

The Couplers

These are simple cavities (either 6 cc or 2 cc) used for the sole purpose of measuring the outputs from earphones (supra-aural, circumaural, and insert) and hearing aids. The two conventional couplers used predominantly for audiometric calibrations are the National Bureau of Standards (NBS) Type 9 A, and the American Standards Association (ASA, now called ANSI) Type 1 couplers as shown in Figure 6–13. The best known of the two and most widely used coupler for audiometric purpose is the NBS Type 9A coupler. These couplers consist of a cylindrical cavity, the base of which is terminated by the diaphragm of the microphone. Both of them are known as 6-cc couplers, because of the amount of air trapped between the microphone and the earphone during measurement. Even though the volume (6 cc) is the same between these couplers, however, their response characteristics differ. The reliability of pressure response of the NBS Type 9A coupler is restricted low frequencies between 0.5 to 1.5 kHz, whereas the ANSI Type 1 couplers produce a constant pressure across frequencies (flat response up to 8.0 kHz) even at the resonant frequency. The reason for this considerable difference for the frequency characteristics is attributed mainly to the difference in their shapes. Given that the Type 1 is technically superior in performance, still it is not as widely used as NBS Type 9A coupler.

The 2-cc coupler on the other hand has been used exclusively for measuring hearing aid electroacoustic characteristics and insert earphones since 1942, and is still used today. These couplers simulate the average ear canal dimensions with an inserted earphone. Currently available 2-cc couplers are HA1, HA2, and HA3; the area in each coupler

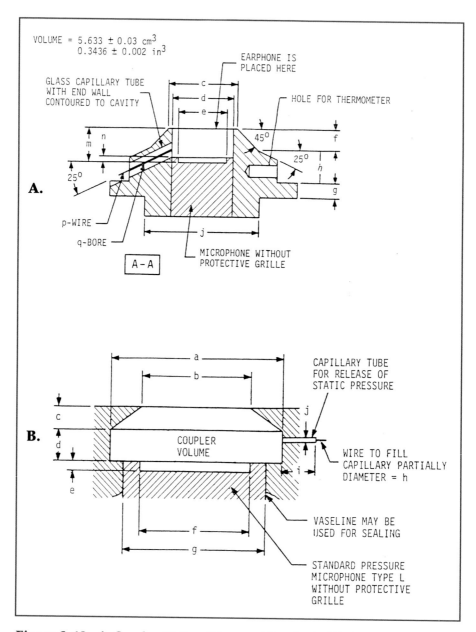

Figure 6–13. **A.** *Couplers National Bureau of Standards (NBS).* **B.** *American Standards Association (ASA or ANSI) Type 1. (Reproduced with permission from American National Standards Institute, New York)*

is adjusted so that the effective volume presented to the microphone is equivalent to 2 cc. The HA-1, illustrated in Figure 6–14, is used for measuring the outputs of in-the-ear hearing aids and insert earphones. The hearing aid or the insert earphone is mounted directly onto the coupler

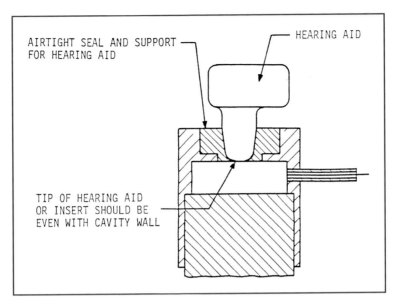

Figure 6–14. *The 2-cm³ couplers: HA-1 used for in-the-ear hearing aid measurements. (ASA or ANSI) Type 1. (Reproduced with permission from American National Standards Institute. New York.)*

using a suitable wax or other type of products to attain an airtight seal around the opening (see Figure 6–14).

The design of the HA-2 is adapted to test the outputs of both body worn hearing aids as shown in Figure 6–15A, as well as the behind-the-ear or eye glass type hearing aids as portrayed in Figure 6–15B. Modifications of HA-2 couplers are designed so that each provides the same 2-cc dimensions required for calibration and measurements. The third coupler, shown in Figure 6–16, is known as the HA-3, which is similar in function to the HA-2 coupler shown in Figure 6–15B; this coupler is designed for better consistency and reproducibility.

Undoubtedly, the 2-cc coupler has been used extensively for measuring hearing aid performance. The use of 2-cc couplers for hearing aid measurements has been questioned, because of the several problems associated with coupler data when compared to a real ear performance. Obviously, the coupler neither simulates the dimensions of adult ear canal nor does it account for the body baffle and head diffraction effects (Muller, Hawkins, & Northern, 1992, p. 4). Another serious concern is that the frequency response of the coupler differs considerably from that of a real ear response. As a result, Beck (1991) pointed out that hearing aid measurement in situ (real-ear) and 2-cc coupler is like speaking in two different languages. Muller et al. stated that, "it is ironic that this 2-cc

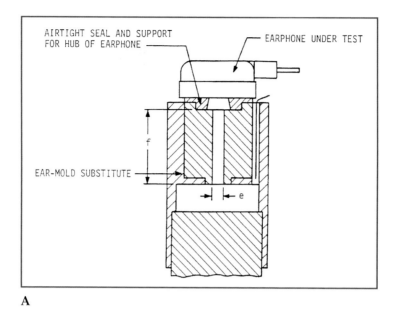

A

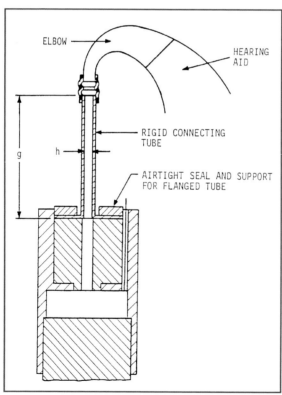

Figure 6–15. *The 2 cm³ couplers.* **A.** *HA-2 coupler used for body type of hearing aid or earphones with snap ring receiver.* **B.** *HA-2 coupler used for behind-the-ear and eye glass type hearing aid measurements (ASA or ANSI) Type1. (Reproduced with permission from American National Standards Institute, New York)*

B

coupler designed as a temporary solution, is still in use nearly 50 years later!" (1992, p. 4). Because of the above reasons probe microphone measurements are gaining considerable popularity as a single most important measuring technique for hearing aid selection and fitting.

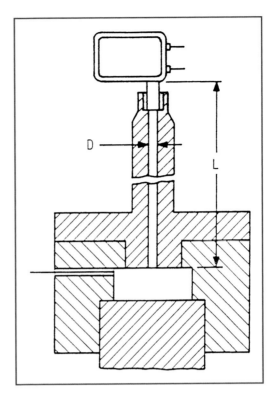

Figure 6–16. *The 2-cm³ couplers. HA-3 (ASA or ANSI) Type 1. (Reproduced with permission from American National Standards Institute, New York)*

The Artificial Ear

The decision to develop an artificial ear was first initiated by the International Electrotechnical Commission (IEC) during 1960. The objective was to construct an artificial ear that matched the impedance of the average human ear. Figure 6–17 illustrates the IEC artificial ear; it consists of three cavities, which are coupled acoustically. This coupler is intended for calibrating supra-aural earphones and not circumaural earphones, and it is designed to cover the frequency range 0.020 kHz to 20.0 kHz. Although IEC 318 artificial ear was an improvement over other couplers, it was still unable to provide the accuracy and consistency needed for many measurements because the geometry of the artificial ear differed considerably from that of a real ear.

The Earlike Coupler

The realistic test of the performance of all these standard couplers including the artificial ear is the quantitative measurement of the amount of pressure developed inside the coupler when compared to a real ear. All

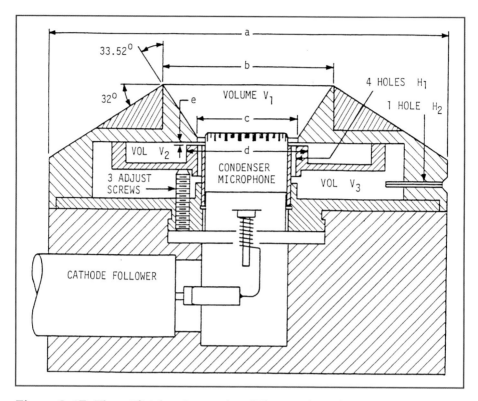

Figure 6–17. *The artificial ear International Electrotechnical Commission (IEC) 318.*

these couplers had shortcomings, because none of them simulated the acoustic impedance of a real ear; as a result the sound pressure measured in the coupler differed substantially from that measured in the real ear. Added to this, earphones matched to produce same output sound pressure level in the real ear, when measured in the couplers produced different sound pressure levels, which explains the need for separate calibration for each earphone used with audiometers. These limitations prompted the searchers to develop a better system that simulated the real ear.

Zwislocki (1971) developed an acoustic coupler known as a "earlike coupler" to overcome the shortcomings and problems of previous couplers. Factors considered for the development of the "earlike coupler" included impedance measurement at the plane of the tympanic membrane and ear, and also considered the average dimensions of the ear canal and concha. The required measurements to develop the earlike coupler was either obtained from several other studies (Delany, 1964; Shaw & Teranishi, 1968; Teranishi & Shaw, 1968) or gathered by Zwislocki (1970, 1971).

The "earlike coupler" diagrammed in Figure 6–18 contains four parts, each part corresponding to an anatomic segment of the outer ear

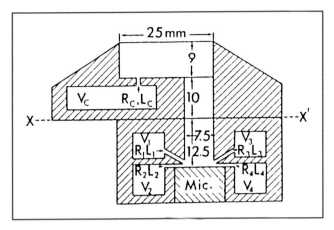

Figure 6–18. *The Zwislocki "Earlike coupler." (Reproduced with permission from Zwislock, 1971)*

(i.e., ear canal and concha), the tympanic membrane, and the head. It contains two sections; the upper part can be used for supra-aural earphones and the lower portion corresponding to the ear canal and the tympanic membrane is suitable for the measurement of insert earphones (Zwislocki, 1971, 1985). The "earlike coupler" has been extensively used for both clinical and research applications and also for the calibration of supra-aural, circumaural, and insert earphones.

The Manikin or KEMAR

The next major development was an effort to produce a realistic manikin to represent the adult anthropomorphic values (Burkhart & Sachs, 1975). Several researchers before Burkhart and Sachs (1975) had tried to provide the dimensions of the human head and body baffle effect; however, due to several design problems most of the earlier models were unsuccessful. The important consideration during the construction of the manikin was to represent an average human adult head and torso dimensions. The manikin constructed by Burkhard and Sachs (1975) is shown in Figure 6–19. Finally, given all the dimensions and factors, the KEMAR was constructed from fiberglass reinforced polyester; considerable attention was given to fabricate the manikin's various dimensions. The Zwislocki "earlike coupler" provided the ear canal and tympanic membrane dimensions and added to the manikin. The manikin reflects human head, torso, and outer ear, as well as fleshlike properties. Finally, the KEMAR was tested for the acoustic properties in a free sound-field; the results between the KEMAR and Shaw's data from humans subjects

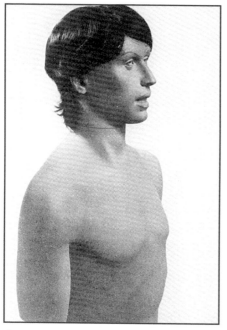
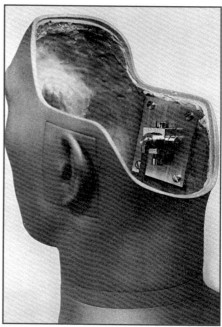

A   B

Figure 6–19. *Manikin or KEMAR (Knowles Electronics Mannikin for Acoustic Research). (Reproduced with permission from Anthropometric Mannikin for Acoustic Research by M. D. Burkhardt and R. M. Sachs, 1975, p. 218.* Journal of Acoustical Society of America, 58. *Copyright 1975 American Institute of Physics)*

are shown in Figure 6–20. Since the introduction of the KEMAR manikin, most precise calibrations are carried out using this instrument. Recently, a smaller manikin was added to simulate a child's head and torso.

Even though the KEMAR provided the important factor to determine the acoustics, still the search for a better system continues. The hearing aid evaluation has finally resolved some of the problems by directly measuring the sound pressure within the ear canal to that of the free-field. The realistic expectation of a coupler would be to provide individual SPL measurements based on the dimensions of each ear canal under test. Even these procedures can be questioned, since the ear canal shape and volume changes due to jaw movements.

Importance of Ear Canal Acoustics in Audiology

In clinical practice, the knowledge of ear canal acoustics is important for two reasons. First, it is important to understand how the sound delivery

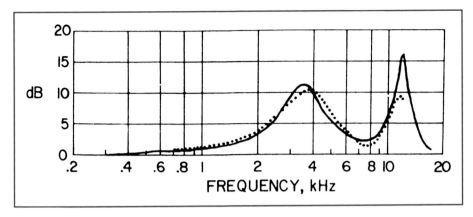

Figure 6–20. *Comparison of sound pressure transfer function from Shaw (1972) and KEMAR data. (Reproduced with permission from Anthropometric Mannikin for Acoustic Research by M. D. Burkhardt and R. M. Sachs, 1975, p. 218. Journal of Acoustical Society of America, 58. Copyright 1975 American Institute of Physics)*

system (i.e., the earphone and hearing aids) and the ear canal can alter the spectral content of the signal reaching the tympanic membrane. Second, the knowledge of ear canal acoustics is important when measuring the sound pressure developed within the canal (i.e., the location of the microphone within the ear canal).

It is crucial to understand what types of sounds are being delivered into the ear canal and to the tympanic membrane during physiologic or behavioral evaluations. Even normal variations in the shape and size of the ear canal can significantly alter the sound pressure buildup within the ear canal. For example, a standard signal such as a click delivered to an adult ear canal may be different from that delivered to an infant's ear canal. Johnson and Nelson (1991) studied acoustic characteristics of clicks routinely used for ABR testing in infants' and adults' ear canals as presented through insert earphones at 30 and 60 dB nHL. The mean resonance frequency recorded for clicks in infants was considerably higher (2339.77 Hz) than in adults (1618.75 Hz). In addition, there was greater variability in the resonance peaks in infants (669.3 Hz) compared to those of adults (319.0 Hz). The differences in the resonant peaks can be attributed to variations in the ear canal dimensions in infants and adults. The spectral differences for clicks in infants should warrant concern when interpreting ABRs or click-evoked otoacoustic emissions (OAEs). According to Rubel, Born, Dietch, and Durham (1984), the responsive region in human neonates is limited to about 500 to 1000 Hz at birth, with increased responsiveness to higher frequencies during the first few months. Therefore, it is likely that the frequency region of a click within the infant's ear canal may be beyond the frequency region capable of exciting a response. This might create reduced excitation of the cochlear region, poor responses, and difficulty in interpreting the test results. Persons concerned with hearing measurements in infants, children, and adults must pay attention to ear canal related variations. Therefore, the importance of individual measurements to determine the type of sound reaching the tympanic membrane must be emphasized in clinical testing.

Hearing aid placement within the canal can also alter the resonance characteristics of the ear canal; the loss of resonance due to placing a hearing aid in the ear canal is known as "insertion loss." Any obstruction in the ear canal (e.g., cerumen or foreign bodies) should be considered during patient testing as a possible source to alter the canal resonance.

In addition, another area that has attracted careful consideration of the ear canal acoustics is in determining the type of sound that reaches the tympanic membrane among individuals exposed to industrial noise. For several years researchers argued that the characteristic 4.0 kHz notch observed in industrial workers exposed to noise was due to susceptibility of the basilar membrane and the middle ear structures. It is interesting to note that individuals exposed to similar types of noises may exhibit differing amounts of hearing loss across frequencies.

Recent findings suggest that the variations in the pattern and magnitude of hearing loss among individuals exposed to similar types of noise may be attributed to differences in the ear canal resonance characteristic of each individual in addition to cochlear susceptibility. Caiazzo and Tonndorf (1977) demonstrated that artificial TTS moved from 4.0 to 2.0 kHz. In another study, Gerhardt, Rodriguez, Helper, and Moul (1987) measured the ear canal pressure distribution for a broadband noise and compared the relationship between TTS and ear canal volume. They reported that subjects with larger ear canal volumes were affected at lower frequencies compared to those with smaller ear canals where maximum TTS was observed at 6.0 kHz. In a later study, Rodriguez and Gerhardt (1991) measured the ear canal resonance and the amount of TTS at different frequencies. The ear canal resonant frequency significantly correlated with the frequency where maximum TTS was observed in 31 of the subjects tested in their study. Even though the relationship between TTS and ear canal resonance is pretty well established, similar relationships between noise-induced hearing loss (NIHL) and resonance characteristics of the ear canal are under study. Additional data from Pierson, Gerhardt, Rodriguez, and Yanke (1994) from 29 patients with positive history of noise exposure and demonstrable hearing loss in the high-frequency regions suggested that there is a high correlation between the ear canal resonance frequency and the audiometric notch.

They concluded that as the peak resonant frequency of the ear canal increased, so did the shift in the frequency of the permanent hearing loss. All these findings clearly suggest that a high degree of relationship exists between the noise-induced hearing loss (NIHL) and ear canal resonance. It should be borne in mind that several factors combine to produce an NIHL; however, the importance of outer ear spectral shaping of a broadband signal should not be ignored.

The second consideration of ear canal acoustics is related to measurements made within the ear canal. Two routine clinical measurements that necessitate probe microphone placement within the ear canal are real ear hearing aid measurement and otoacoustic emission testing. In both these tests the reliability and accuracy of the measurement depends on the location of the probe tube/microphone. To improve the reliability of these measurements (especially real ear hearing aid measurements), the microphone/probe tube placement should be close to the tympanic membrane without causing any discomfort to the patient.

Summary

In many cases the ear canal has been treated as a straight tube of uniform cross-section with the tympanic membrane terminating the tube perpendicularly. With this model, the prediction of sound pressure within the ear canal is quite accurate up to 4.0 to 8.0 kHz. However, at higher frequencies (i.e., greater than 8.0 kHz), the above model fails to predict the pressure distribution because of intersubject differences in canal geometry and consequent variations in the acoustical transformation between the sound-field and tympanic membrane. These individual differences will undoubtedly influence the outcome of various clinical, psychoacoustic, and physiologic studies in humans and in animals. In addition, knowledge of ear canal geometry due to variations caused by factors like jaw movement is important when fitting hearing aids. Furthermore, knowledge of ear canal variations between children and adults are important for understanding the directional sensitivity of sound pressure in localization function, and in determining temporary or permanent threshold shifts.

7

Deep Canal Hearing Aids

BRIAN TAYLOR

The external auditory canal is an important factor in any hearing aid fitting, as the canal directs amplified sound toward the tympanic membrane. In the case of many deep canal fittings, however, the external auditory canal also serves as the location for the hearing instrument itself. Regardless of the specific type of hearing aid fitting, the external ear canal plays three significant roles in the fitting of hearing aids. One, it serves to direct amplified sound toward the tympanic membrane. Two, the ear canal shapes incoming sound by acting as a resonator. Three, it assists in holding the earmold or custom-made device securing within the ear.

Because the ear canal is a dynamic part of the human anatomy, special attention must always be taken when fitting hearing aids. This care and attention takes on even greater importance when fitting deep canal instruments. There are several aspects to fitting deep canal hearing aids that are unique and different relative to other types of hearing aids fittings. Selection criteria, impression taking, gain requirements, and patient benefits are among the differences that must be considered when selecting and fitting deep canal devices. Many of these considerations are addressed in detail in this chapter.

A deep canal hearing aid is defined as any device that terminates beyond the second bend of the ear canal within 5 mm of the tympanic membrane. A deep canal fitting can be accomplished with any hearing aid or earmold in which the eartip extends into the bony portion of the ear canal. Figure 7–1 shows two distinctly different styles of hearing aids that are both deep canal devices.

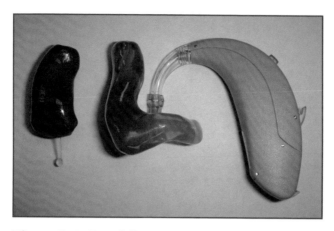

Figure 7–1. *Two different styles of deep canal fittings. The completely-in-the-canal (CIC) is on the left and the behind-the-ear (BTE) is on the right.*

The term "deep canal" refers to the place where the instrument ends in the ear canal, not to a particular style of hearing aid. On the other hand, completely-in-the-canal (CIC), mini CIC, invisible-in-the-canal (IIC) peritympanic, and "extended wear" instruments are different types of styles or form factors which place the microphone at least 1 to 2 mm beyond the opening of the ear canal and require a deep canal fitting. To be classified as a deep canal instrument it is essential that the eartip of the device terminates beyond the second bend and makes contact with the bony portion of the external auditory canal. This is illustrated by the device on the right-hand side in Figure 7–1. Notice that both devices are CICs; however, only the CIC on the right-hand side of Figure 7–2 is considered a deep canal fitting. This chapter primarily focuses on deep canal fittings in which both the microphone and receiver are located beyond the opening of the ear canal, like the deep canal CIC in Figure 7–2.

History of Deep Fitting Canal Hearing Aids

Over the past few decades, the popularity of deep canal hearing instruments has ebbed and flowed. The first documented case of the use of a deep canal fitting was in the mid-1970s (Bolger et al., 1975). Referred to as an "auriculostomy" this deep canal application isolated the receiver of the hearing into an earmold embedded as deeply as possible in the ear canal. The deep canal fitting resulted in reports of minimal occlusion, better speech understanding, and improved sound quality.

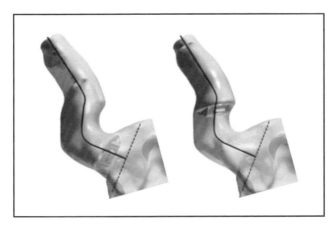

Figure 7–2. *Two different completely-in-the-canal (CIC) products. The deep canal CIC is on the right. Images provided by Starkey Laboratories, Inc. Reprinted with permission.*

In the late 1980s deep canal fittings resurfaced as a viable alternative for adult patients with severe hearing loss who wanted to wear their hearing aids during recreational activities. Full shell and behind-the-ear instruments were manufactured with extended canal lengths in order to provide adequate gain and output while minimizing acoustic feedback. Similar instruments with long canal lengths also began to be used as part of a transcranial CROS arrangement (Staab, 1989). At about this same time some hearing care professionals began to tout the added benefits of reduced occlusion and the high frequency gain advantages of a deep fitting instrument (Killion et al., 1988).

In the early 1990s Philips Hearing Instruments introduced the XP peritympanic hearing instrument. Some of the unique features of the peritympanic CIC instrument included a special impression-taking technique with aeration tubes as part of the otoblock, a removal cord and soft tip on the instrument, and routine use of video-otoscopy during the impression-taking process. These techniques and equipment, associated with the use of the peritympanic CIC were incorporated into the completely-in-the-canal (CIC), which became very popular in the early to mid 1990s. By having a shorter, tapered canal length and requiring a less invasive ear impression procedure, the CIC differed in a couple of important ways from the peritympanic CIC. Given its cosmetic appeal, ease of use on the phone and other inherent acoustic advantages, the CIC style enjoyed approximately 15% of the total hearing instrument market share in the late 1990s.

During the 2000s the open canal BTE instrument became available and some of the patient advantages from CICs, including reduction in occlusion and cosmetic appeal now existed in another style, and the popularity of the CIC waned. Although the CIC has lost market share over the past 15 years, deep canal fittings have not been abandoned. Recently, several manufacturers have introduced new styles of deep canal devices, including extended wear instruments, micro CIC, and invisible-in-the-canal (IIC) products. Regardless of the specific name, all of these devices require a deep fitting canal. With improvements in impression taking equipment, miniaturization of digital signal processing and the patient benefits associated with deep canal instruments, these devices are beginning to enjoy resurgence in popularity. This chapter next evaluates the benefits of deep canal fittings.

The Acoustics of Deep Canal Hearing Aids

Specific benefits of deep canal hearing aids, which terminate within the bony structure of the ear canal, have been well known for quite some time (Bryant et al., 1982; Staab, 1993; Staab & Finlay, 1991; Varoba, 1987). Although deep canal fittings are often associated with CIC style devices, many of the acoustic advantages discussed in this chapter also apply to other hearing aid styles, such as full shell ITEs that have a long canal extending beyond the second bend of the ear canal. To better appreciate the acoustics of deep canal hearing aids, the reader needs a clear understanding of how deep canal fittings differ from BTE, ITE, and other types of fittings with shorter canal lengths. A good starting point of these important differences begins with a review of Boyle's law.

Boyle's law, which was first published in 1660, describes the inverse relationship between the volume and pressure of a gas within a closed system. In the case of a hearing aid fitting, the "closed system" is the space between the tympanic membrane (TM) and the end of the hearing aid, the "volume" is the space between the TM and the hearing aid, and the "pressure" is the intensity of the sound generated by the device. A deep canal fitting decreases the volume of the air between the TM and hearing aid, which results in a significant increase in sound pressure level. The inverse relationship that exists between volume and pressure results in a sound energy increase of approximately 10 to 15 dB (Chasin, 1995). In essence, as the eartip of the instrument is pushed closer to the TM, thus reducing the volume of air, the sound pressure increases in a systematic manner.

Compared to the 2-cc coupler, the equivalent ear canal volume of the human ear is 1.26 cc (ANSI S3.25). When the eartip of any hearing instrument is extended into the ear canal, the equivalent ear canal volume is reduced to approximately 0.4 cc. Therefore, Boyle's law indicates a gain improvement of approximately 10 dB, which is derived from 20 log 10(1.26 cc/0.4 cc) simply reducing the volume of the closed ear canal.

Because the ear canal is not a hard-walled cavity this calculation is not quite as straightforward on actual ears. As the ear canal consists of living tissue (and not a hard-walled cavity); the change in sound pressure is about 5 dB in the low frequencies and between 9 and 12 dB for the high frequencies (Staab, 1997). When fitting any hearing aid there are differences between the output of the hearing aid in the hard-walled 2-cc coupler and the human ear that warrant further explanation. In case of deep canal fittings, these differences are more pronounced, as illustrated in Figure 7–3.

As previously mentioned most deep canal fittings place the microphone at least 1–2 mm beyond the opening of the ear canal; therefore, there are two other acoustical differences that must be considered relative to behind-the-ear (BTE) and other types of larger in-the-ear (ITE) instruments of the deep canal variety. The concha-related Helmholtz resonance is 6 to 8 dB in magnitude and is typically found between 4000 and 5000 Hz. In a deep canal CIC device the sound energy is enhanced by the concha-related resonance before it enters the microphone of the hearing aid. Chasin (1995) refers to this as the "pop bottle" resonance because it is created by similar physics as the sound one hears when

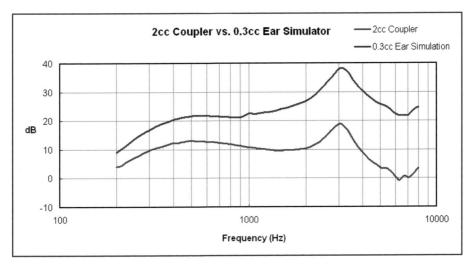

Figure 7–3. *The frequency response of a typical deep canal fitting (top curve) in a 0.3-cc ear simulator compared to a more conventional fitting (lower curve) in a 2-cc coupler.*

one blows across the top of a pop bottle. Figure 7–4 shows the effect of the concha-related Helmholtz resonance for KEMAR compared to a real person. This can be done using standard probe microphone equipment and conducting a REUR measure with the concha occluded with putty. Note in this example that the concha-related resonance is much greater for KEMAR than the individual.

Another important resonator is the so-called pinna effect. The pinna effect is a high frequency enhancement of sound energy due to the shorter wavelengths of sound energy reflecting off the surface of the pinna. As sound energy is being reflected like a mirror off the pinna, Chasin (1995) refers to the pinna effect as "the mirror." Due to their shorter wavelengths, lower frequencies (1000 Hz or less) pass through the pinna unaffected. The pinna effect occurs above 2000 Hz and increases with frequency. Figure 7–5 shows the pinna effect for three different microphone locations.

Given that the microphone of a deep canal instrument can be several millimeters from the opening of the ear canal, the combined effects of the pinna effect and concha-related resonance can be as large as 8 dB in the high frequencies (Preves, 1994). Thus, the combined effects of a deeply placed receiver and microphone result in about a 5 dB increase in sound energy for low frequencies (250 to 750 Hz) and a 12 to 17 dB increase in high frequency energy (Arbogast & Whichard, 2009; Chasin,

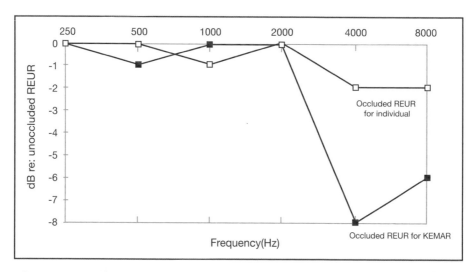

Figure 7–4. *Effects of occluding the concha on KEMAR and one individual's ear referenced according to the unoccluded real-ear unaided response (REUR). (From The Acoustic Advantages of CIC Hearing Aids by M. Chasin, 1994, p. 13,* Hearing Journal, 47 *(11). Copyright 1994 by Williams & Wilins Publishing Company. Reprinted by permission.)*

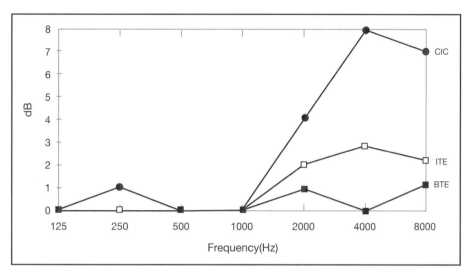

Figure 7–5. *The pinna effect for three different microphone locations: behind-the-ear (BTE), in-the-ear (ITE), and completely-in-the canal (CIC). (From The Acoustic Advantages of CIC Hearing Aids by M. Chasin, 1994, p. 14. Hearing Journal, 47(11). Copyright 1994 by Williams & Wilkins Publishing Company. Reprinted by permission.)*

1995; Gudmundsen, 1994). Let's turn our attention to how these differences relate to fitting hearing aids in real ears.

In order to better understand how the acoustics of deep canal CIC fittings differ with other types of styles of hearing aids, it helps to review three correction factors: the CORFIG, the TEREO and the RECD, and how these correction factors vary across hearing aid styles. (There's a lot to know about the CORFIG, TEREO, and RECD and the interested reader is encouraged to check out some of the references listed in this section to learn more about correction factors.)

As previously mentioned (see Figure 7–3), there are significant differences between gain in a 2-cc coupler and the human ear, which must be considered. These differences in gain and output also vary as a function of hearing aid style. The coupler response for flat insertion gain (CORFIG), which takes into account microphone location effects (MLE), the real ear to coupler difference (RECD), and the individual's real ear unaided response (REUR), is used to calculate the difference in gain between the 2-cc coupler and the actual ear. Because the MLE (Figure 7–6) varies across hearing aid styles, the CORFIG is different for deep canal CIC fittings compared to other styles.

Table 7–1 shows the CORFIG values used for four different types of hearing aid styles. In order to obtain an estimation of real ear gain, these CORFIG values need to be added to the 2-cc coupler values. Or, when

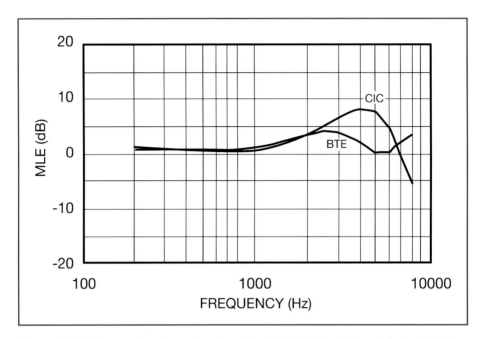

Figure 7–6. *Mean microphone location effects (MLEs) for CIC and for behind-the-ear instruments (Bentler & Pavlovic, 1989) measured at 0° azimuth.*

Table 7–1. CORFIG Values for Four Different Styles of Hearing Aids

Frequency (Hz)	250	500	1000	2000	4000	8000
BTE	−4	−2	0	−1	−5	1
ITE	−1	−2	1	0	2	11
ITC	−1	−2	1	0	5	13
CIC	7	7	9	7	18	23

Source: Macrae and Dillon (1996). *Journal of Rehabilitation Research and Development, 33*(4), 235.

ordering hearing aids, the values in Table 7–1 would be subtracted from the desired real ear insertion gain (REIG) to obtain the 2-cc coupler targets.

Today, insertion gain measures aren't nearly as popular as they were when deep canal CICs were introduced on the market in the mid 1990s. The real-ear aided response (REAR) is a more common measure of hearing aid performance. In order to transform the 2-cc coupler measure to the REAR, the TEREO is needed. TEREO stands for transform for estimating real ear output, and it is comprised of the MLE and RECD. For example, the TEREO would be subtracted from the REAR to obtain the equivalent 2-cc coupler values. Or, if you already have the 2-cc coupler values, you would add the TEREO to predict the REAR.

The TEREO and CORFIG are used to convert 2-cc coupler to real ear *gain* measures. On the other hand the real ear to coupler difference (RECD), which has already been mentioned a couple of times in this chapter is used to convert output in the 2-cc coupler to output in the ear. As you might have guessed, there are some important differences in output in a deep canal fit compared to other fittings and the RECD can help us understand those differences (see Seewald et al., 1995, for more information on the TEREO and CORFIG).

In order to better understand the unique gain requirements of a deep canal fitting relative to other fittings, let's work through an example using one of the transfer functions. Let's say your afternoon patient has a flat 40 dB hearing loss and he wants a deep canal CIC device. You enter these thresholds into your favorite prescriptive fitting formula and it gives you specific gain targets for each frequency, using the CORFIG you quickly find the target 2-cc coupler gain needed for this hearing loss. After factoring in the reserve gain, you have the amount of required gain (this is in bold in Table 7–2). The 2-cc coupler required gain for the deep canal CIC fitting is compared to a typical ITE fitting. Notice that in order to match the REIG target for this hearing loss, the ITE requires 20 dB or more gain at some frequencies. It's from these differences in transfer

Table 7–2. Calculations for Transforming the Desired REIG to the Desired 2-cc Coupler Response for a CIC Compared to an ITE

Frequency (Hz)	250	500	1000	2000	4000	6000
Target REIG	1	10	19	17	16	16
(+) CORFIG	–7	–7	–9	–7	–18	–23
Target 2-cc User Gain	–6	3	10	10	–2	–7
Reserve Gain	10	10	10	10	10	10
Target 2-cc FOG (CIC)	4	13	20	20	8	3
Target 2-cc FOG (ITE)	10	18	30	27	28	36
CIC/ITE Difference	6	5	10	7	20	33

functions between the CIC and the ITE (bottom line of Table 7–2, also in bold) that should help you understand that for the same hearing loss, you need *less* gain from the CIC to match a prescriptive formula.

It is unlikely that you will have to ever make a CORFIG, TEREO or RECD calculation in your head (fitting software and probe microphone equipment often do it automatically), but a good understanding of these transfer functions helps to understand the acoustical differences between deep canal fittings relative to other types of fittings. It is this difference that forms the basis for many of the advantages of deep canal CIC instruments.

Benefits of Deep Canal Fittings

All of the acoustical characteristics of deep canal fittings that were explored in the previous section offer patients some unique benefits relative to other types of fittings. The expected patient benefits of placing the microphone and receiver closer to the tympanic membrane offer many potential advantages, including improved headroom, increased high frequency gain, and fewer problems with feedback. The potential benefits of deep canal fittings are covered in this section.

Less Gain and Output Needed to Provide Audibility

Given the difference is microphone and receiver location compared to other fittings, deep canal devices less 2-cc coupler gain is required relative to other fittings to fit the same hearing loss. This point is illustrated in Table 7–2. As pushing the microphone and receiver closer to the tympanic membrane results in the need for less gain, the fitting range of deep canal instruments can be expanded. In other words, deep canal instruments can often provide sufficient audibility for moderate to severe high-frequency hearing losses.

Increased High Frequency Gain

The combination of deeper microphone and receiver placement results in 12 to 17 dB in additional high frequency gain. Therefore, a deep fitting instrument has the potential to provide greater amounts of high frequency gain with *less* output from the hearing aid amplifier. In addition to providing adequate high frequency gain to restore audibility, another potential benefit of deep fitting devices is they can be used effectively for precipitous hearing frequency losses (Gudmundsen, 1994).

When a deep canal instrument is tightly sealed into the bony portion of the ear canal, higher amounts of gain and output can be delivered without feedback. Subsequently, the SSPL-90 output and 2-cc gain sufficient for a 55 to 60 dB high frequency hearing loss with a typical BTE or custom ITE would be adequate for a 70 to 75 dB high frequency loss with a deep fitting CIC. An obvious implication is that audibility can be restored for more severe hearing loss by providing less gain and output from a deep fitting instrument.

Increased Undistorted Output (headroom)

Hearing aid headroom is identified as the difference between the output of the hearing aid (input plus gain) and the SSPL90. Compared to traditional hearing aids, deep canal hearing aid fittings require less output when fitting the same hearing loss. As less output is needed to make sounds sufficiently audible for the patient, the hearing aid amplifier is less likely to be driven into saturation, where audible distortion can occur. This often leads to an increase in hearing aid headroom. Expanding hearing aid headroom is identified as contributing significantly to hearing aid quality (Preves & Woodruff, 1990). Additionally, an increase in hearing aid headroom allows for greater output in a hearing aid without reaching the aided loudness discomfort level of the patient (Fortune & Preves, 1992).

Reduced Occlusion Effect

The occlusion effect can be best described as an echo or hollow sensation occurring when the patient is speaking or chewing. Older patients often describe it as sounding like they are "talking in a barrel" (young people don't talk in barrels so much) "my voice is too loud" or "hollow sounding voice." This sensation can be highly annoying and it is more likely to occur with patients having better than 30 to 40 dB HL thresholds in the low frequencies.

When we talk, sound energy from vocalizations in the back of our throat travels to the ear canal through via bone conduction through the mandible (jawbone). Bone-conducted sound causes the cartilaginous portion of the ear-canal to vibrate, which creates an air conduction sound in the ear canal (primarily low frequency). Normally, this sound energy escapes through the open ear. But if the ear canal is closed off by the hearing aid shell or earmold, the energy is transferred through the middle ear to the cochlea. Thus, the patient with this problem often complains that their own voice sounds loud, hollow (because it primarily enhances the low frequencies) or unusual when they talk. With some probe-mic equipment, you can attach earphones, and listen to this yourself from your patient's ear.

By sealing the earmold or shell beyond the second bend of the ear canal, the vibration of the cartilaginous portion of the canal is held to a minimum and problems associated with the occlusion effect are minimized. For this reason, an advantage of a deep canal instrument is a reduction in problems associated with the occlusion effect.

Reduction in Feedback

Acoustic feedback (i.e., squealing) is an extremely annoying problem for some hearing aid users. Feedback is directly related to the amount of gain needed to restore audibility and the size of the hearing aid vent. As a deep canal fitting requires less gain relative to a fitting with a traditional canal length for the same hearing loss, feedback may be less problematic. Recently, automatic feedback cancellation systems have been introduced to the market that allows the hearing aid to provide more gain without feedback. To date, results of these automatic feedback cancellers have been mixed. In addition to the gain requirements of the device, the effectiveness of feedback cancellers is dependent on the geometry of the ear canal and the integrity of the feedback cancellation algorithm (Ricketts et al., 2008). Although some feedback cancellers have been shown to provide over 15 dB of added gain before feedback when they are activated, they sometimes introduce audible distortions (i.e., entrainment) which can result in poor sound quality.

As a deep canal instrument provides a tight seal in the bony portion of the ear canal, occlusion problems are minimized without the use of venting. Consequently, reliance on feedback cancelation algorithms to eliminate acoustic feedback may be reduced with some deep canal fittings.

Natural Directionality and Localization

Recall that the ear canal, concha and pinna all play integral roles in filtering sound energy before it reaches the tympanic membrane. These anatomical landmarks of the outer ear are important for localization. Depending on the microphone location of the hearing aid, the ability of these landmarks to localize sounds are completely lost or minimized. Deep canal fittings have been shown to retain some aspects of the ears' natural ability to localize sounds as compared to a BTE instrument. Figure 7–7 shows three measurements of the directivity index: a completely open unaided ear, a deep canal instrument and a BTE hearing aid. Results of the deep canal instrument show directionality very similar to the open ear. The data in Figure 7–7 suggest that deep canal instruments will provide improved localization ability when compared to a BTE hearing aid fitting (Best et al., 2010).

Ease of Use With Telephones/Cell Phones

Telephone use is one of the most critical listening areas for many hearing aid users (Kochkin, 2010). Because the microphone of most deep canal instrument is located at least 1 to 2 mm beyond the opening of the ear canal, many patients can place the handset of a landline telephone or cell phone up to their ear without feedback or discomfort. This can provide a significant ease of use advantage for individuals who spend a lot of time talking on the telephone.

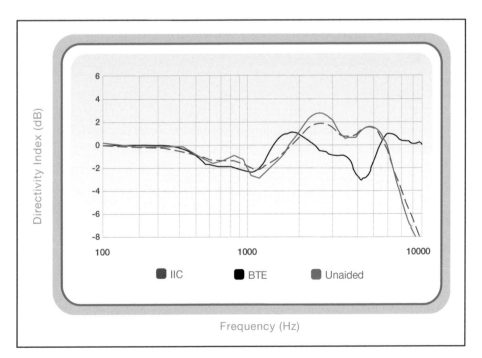

Figure 7–7. *KEMAR based measurements of directivity comparing the open ear (unaided) to a BTE and invisible-in-the-canal (deep canal) fitting. Provided by Starkey Laboratories, Inc. Reprinted with permission.*

Wind Noise

Amplification of wind noise is often problematic for hearing aid users. In fact, most manufacturers use special noise reduction algorithms to reduce wind noise and its deleterious effects. Deep canal fittings offer an alternative to wind noise reduction algorithms since the microphone on most deep canal products is located beyond the opening of the ear canal. As a general rule, the deeper the microphone is located within the ear canal, the less interference of amplified sound caused by wind noise.

Nonacoustic Benefits of Deep Canal Instruments

In addition to the acoustic advantages of deep canal instruments there are other potential benefits associated with their use.

- *Physical Comfort.* For the appropriate candidate, given adequate time to adjust to the initial fitting, deep canal devices have been reported to be extremely comfortable (Gudmundsen, 1994). Recently, introduced deep canal extended wear devices have been reported to be worn comfortably by patients for as long as four months (Scherl et al., 2011).

- *Cosmetics.* Stigma associated with hearing loss and aging continues to plague the profession of audiology. When deep canal CIC and peritympanic devices became popular in the mid 1990s it was thought user acceptance and market penetration would improvement. Unfortunately, the negative affects of stigma remained essentially unchanged almost two decades after these devices came to market. With the recent introduction of extended wear deep canal devices, market penetration and user acceptance have the potential to improve. Given their essentially invisible appearance, recent developments in deep canal devices may have the potential to broaden the market of hearing aid users.

- *Practice Economics.* In addition to all the benefits listed here, deep canal instruments offer a cosmetically appealing alternative to other hearing aids on the market today. A recent study by Arbogast (2010a) indicated that one extended-wear deep canal device attracted new patients to a practice who ordinarily would not have sought consult for their hearing loss. From an economic standpoint deep canal devices offer an alternative source of patients for a practice.

Clinical Considerations

There are several factors that must be evaluated prior to fitting a deep canal instrument for a patient. Without ample consideration of these factors, deep canal fittings are likely to result poor patient outcomes, may put the patient at risk for medical complications. These factors are reviewed in this section.

Candidacy

Not all patients are viable candidates for deep canal instruments. Proper candidate selection must occur during the prefitting process and falls into six main categories: communication needs, lifestyle, audiometric results, medical history, ear canal geometry, and expectations. This section of the chapter addresses how candidacy requirements differ in deep canal fittings relative to other types of fittings.

For any hearing aid candidate communication needs must be assessed during the pre-fitting appointment. Assessment tools such as the COSI (Dillon et al., 1997) or TELEGRAM (Thibodeau, 2004) can be used to measure degree of communication difficulty. Given the fact that current deep fitting instruments don't offer telecoils, directional microphones or easy access to on-board manual control they may not be the best choice for some patients, depending on the communication needs of the individual. On the other hand, deep canal instruments have some inherent ease of use advantages that must be discussed with the patient.

Patient lifestyle is another important pre-fitting consideration. As many clinicians know from experience, patients with a more active lifestyle have a tendency to desire the cosmetic appearance of deep canal instruments. Patients who have been successful with deep canal products come from all walks of life and range in age from nine to 100 (Arbogast, 2010b). One way to determine if cosmetic appearance is a strong motivator for the patient would be to administer the Characteristics of Amplification Tool (COAT) during the prefitting process. The COAT (Sandridge & Newman, 2006) questionnaire, which is shown in Figure 7–8, has the potential to systematically assist clinicians and patients in determining hearing aid feature priorities. Specifically, questions five and six of the COAT are helpful for identifying good deep canal candidates from a lifestyle and patient preference standpoint. For example, if results of the COAT suggest cosmetics are a high priority, then the patient may be a stronger candidate for a deep canal product.

Characteristics of Amplification Tool (COAT)

Name: _____   Date: _____

Our goal is to maximize your ability to hear so that you can more easily communicate with others. In order to reach this goal, it is important that we understand your communication needs, your personal preferences, and your expectations. By having a better understanding of your needs, we can use our expertise to recommend the hearing aids that are most appropriate for **you**. By working together **we** will find the best solution for you.

Please complete the following questions. Be as honest as possible. Be as precise as possible. Thank you.

1.   Please list the top three situations where you would most like to hear better. Be as specific as possible.

    _____

    _____

    _____

2.   How important is it for you to hear better? Mark an X on the line.

    Not Very Important   --   *Very Important*

3.   How motivated are you to wear and use hearing aids? Mark an X on the line.

    Not Very Motivated   --   *Very Motivated*

4.   How well do you think hearing aids will improve your hearing? Mark an X on the line.

    I expect them to:

    Not be helpful   --   *Greatly improve*
    at all   *my hearing*

5.   What is your most important consideration regarding hearing aids? Rank order the following factors with **1** as the most important and **4** as the least important. Place an **X** on the line if the item has no importance to you at all.

    ____   Hearing aid size and the ability of others not to see the hearing aids

    ____   Improved ability to hear and understand speech

    ____   Improved ability to understand speech in noisy situations (e.g., restaurants, parties)

    ____   Cost of the hearing aids

6.   Do you prefer hearing aids that: (check one)

    ____   are totally automatic so that you do not have to make any adjustments to them.
    ____   allow you to adjust the volume and change the listening programs as you see fit.
    ____   no preference

7.   How confident do you feel that you will be successful in using hearing aids.

    Not Very Confident   --   *Very Confident*

Figure 7–8. *The COAT is a prefitting questionnaire that can be administered to the patient before their hearing aid evaluation. Reprinted with the permission of the authors.*

Deep canal devices can accommodate a wide range of hearing losses. Both the degree of hearing loss and slope of the audiogram are important considerations that were discussed earlier in this chapter. The shaded area in Figure 7–9 suggests that mild to severe hearing losses can be fitted with deep canal devices. In Figure 7–9 note the white line running between 60 dB HL in the low frequencies to 70 dB in the high frequencies. As a general rule, deep canal devices provide adequate amounts of gain for hearing losses above this white line in Figure 7–9. Fitting guidelines and gain requirements do vary depending on the specific deep canal product and model. Therefore, clinicians should check with individual manufacturers for more specific information. Clinicians also should be mindful of the fact that the manufacturer's fitting guidelines and gain requirements are merely suggestions, as prescriptive fitting targets and probe microphone measures should be used whenever possible in the fitting process in order to individualize gain, output and the frequency response to the patient.

As deep canal devices fit in the sensitive bony portion of the ear canal, some patients with medical conditions may be precluded from

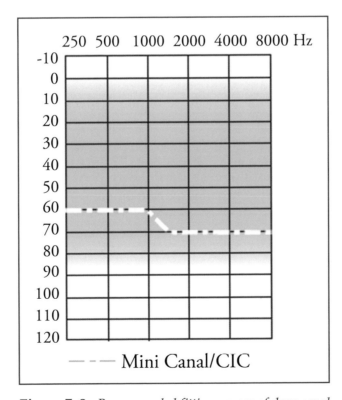

Figure 7–9. *Recommended fitting ranges of deep canal CIC instrument.*

using them. During the prefitting appointment it is imperative for clinicians to carefully evaluate this aspect of candidacy and involve physicians when necessary.

During the otoscopic examination the ear canal must be carefully evaluated. Patients who have an ear canal that has a healthy appearance would be considered candidates for deep canal products. Patients with extremely thin or dry skin in the ear canal are not considered good candidates. Medical conditions, such as osteomas, chronic or recurrent otitis externa, excessive cerumen, and other skin conditions are not viable candidates for deep canal products. Middle ear conditions, such as tympanic membrane perforation, cholesteatoma, use of pressure-equalization tubes and chronic otorrhea are also not considered good candidates.

Medical conditions such as TMJ disorder, otalgia, use of anticoagulation medications, uncontrolled diabetes, immune disorders, and history of radiation therapy to the head or neck as well as chemotherapy within the past year are considered contraindications for use of a deep canal device. Care must be taken during the case history to ensure that all these conditions are discussed with the patient and recorded in the patient's chart notes. Additionally, medical approval from a physician, preferably an otolaryngologist is recommended prior to fitting a deep canal device.

The geometry or shape of the ear canal is another important prefitting consideration. During the prefitting otoscopic examination, the clinician must evaluate the ear canal and ensure that it is not too narrow or too short. Other less common contraindications related to ear canal geometry include a significant step-up in the canal floor, extreme V-shaped canal, a tortuous canal bend, or a large bulge in the canal. These contraindications increase the chance of discomfort when wearing a deep canal instrument and may result in a rejection of the product by the patient.

Proper expectations of deep canal device performance and benefit need to be aligned with the patient. Given the somewhat invasive nature of deep canal devices, some discomfort during their initial use should be expected. This expectation needs to be clearly communicated to the patient.

Prefitting Issues

In addition to assessing patient candidacy, there are several other issues that must be evaluated during the prefitting consultation prior to use of any deep canal instrument. The issues listed below are not unique to deep canal fittings, but due to the depth of fitting special consideration is warranted.

Visualization of the Ear Canal

Examination of the entire ear canal is critically important during the pre-fitting stages of deep canal product use. Examination of the ear canal must be made with a good quality otoscope or a medical microscope. Otoscopy enables that clinician to evaluate the overall health of the ear canal, assess the shape of the ear canal, and determine if cerumen will be an issue relative to candidacy.

Impression Taking

For deep canal devices requiring a custom fit, an ear impression is needed. An ear impression for a customized deep canal device must extend 9 to 12 mm beyond the second bend of the ear canal. Any ear impression puts the patient in some degree of risk; however, because of the extremely long nature of the impression required for a deep canal fit, the risk factor is higher. Thus, safety of the patient must be the highest priority. Good visualization of the ear canal using a high quality otoscope or micro-scope is needed. No special ear impression material is typically required relative to other types of custom devices. Silicone impression material with a high flow and low viscosity is usually recommended; however, you must check with the specific manufacturer of the deep canal device prior to taking any impressions for it.

After completing the patient history and otoscopy, a flattened vented cotton oto-dam, similar to the one in Figure 7–10, is placed deep

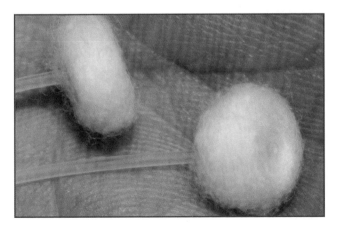

Figure 7–10. *Two vented cotton oto-dams used to make ear impressions for custom-made deep canal devices. Provided by Starkey Laboratories, Inc. Reprinted with permission.*

in the ear canal within 3 to 4 mm of the tympanic membrane. Some clinicians prefer to use a microphone to ensure the oto-dam is properly placed. Proper placement of the oto-dam is shown in Figure 7–11. The clinician must always check with an otoscope or microscope to ensure the flattened cotton oto-dam is completely blocking the tympanic membrane. The oto-dam can be lubricated with Oto-Ease or a similar material to improve comfort while placing it deep in the ear canal. Other aspects of impression taking are similar to traditional customized hearing aids.

Comfort of Fit

As a deep canal instrument is making contact with the bony portion of the ear canal, which is extremely sensitive, physical comfort is a primary consideration. The overall comfort of the deep canal fit is related to the following: (1) the physical comfort of the hearing aid in the ear canal; (2) the sensation of fullness in the ear; and (3) the feeling of pressure within the ear.

The external one-third to one-half of the external canal has a skin lining about 0.5 to 1.0 mm thick, along with a well-developed subcutaneous layer. The result is that this portion of the ear canal is rather forgiving of imperfections in the hearing aid, which may result from a less

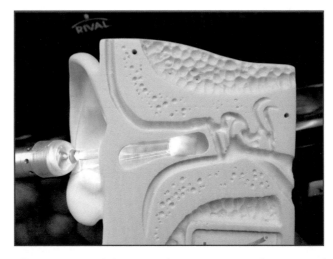

Figure 7–11. *Schematic showing proper placement of the otodam prior to taking an ear impression for a deep canal instrument. Provided by Starkey Laboratories, Inc. Reprinted with permission.*

than perfect ear impression. On the other hand, the internal one-half to two-thirds of the external ear canal has a skin thickness of approximately 0.2 mm and has no subcutaneous layer. Very minor size and shape deviations in the hearing from the ear impression can cause irritation and discomfort while wearing the hearing aid.

Another factor that can result in discomfort associated with deep canal fittings is related to jaw movement. The movement of the condyloid process of the ramus of the mandible in relation to the ear canal varies over a rather wide range. The mandible moves in three axes of rotation: vertical, horizontal, rotational (Edwards & Harris, 1990). When hearing aids extend deeply into the ear canal jaw movement can cause discomfort unless the hearing aid is made from a soft flexible material. Even for some patients, soft shells will result in comfort problems (Staab, 1995).

Due to size constraints, deep canal fittings have extremely small pressure or trench vent. Lybarger (1978) has suggested that a vent as small as 0.025 inches (0.635 mm) will sufficiently allow for pressure equalization. However, some deep canal fittings do not have any venting. As a result, a sensation of pressure or fullness in the ear may occur. This pressure or fullness in the ear should not be confused with the occlusion effect, which we discussed earlier in this chapter. With effective counseling, correct candidacy selection and the use of proper ear impression techniques, discomfort, pressure, and fullness will be minimized.

Cerumen-Related Problems

Another important prefitting consideration of deep canal devices is cerumen causing damage to the receiver of the hearing aid. The leading cause of hearing aid repairs is damage to the receiver, which is usually cause by immersion of the eartip of the hearing aid in the cerumen of the ear canal. In theory, deep canal placement of the receiver, beyond the cerumen production area of the ear canal, minimizes these types of problems. However, in practice, deep canal users can still be plagued with cerumen plugging the receiver opening. Because of deep canal fittings must be pushed through the cartilaginous part of the ear canal, where cerumen is produced, these patients are often prone to cerumen related receiver damage. Patients with excessive cerumen buildup should be discouraged from using deep canal devices that require daily insertion of the device through the ear canal.

Fitting and Follow-Up

The fitting appointment for a patient being fitted with deep canal instruments is similar to any other device with a few exceptions. In addition to ensuring the deep canal device fits properly and the patient is orientated to it as needed, it is recommended that the gain and output of the device is individualized to the patient using a prescriptive formula, such the NAL-NL2 or DSL-I/O v.5 for adults. Verification of the prescriptive formula can be conducted with probe microphone measures.

Although it is recommended that you place the tip of the probe tube 5 mm beyond the tip of the hearing aid, this rule does not apply for deep canal instruments. For deep canal fittings it is recommended that the probe tube is 1 to 2 mm beyond the tip of the hearing aid (Mueller & Hall, 1998). In some cases insertion of the probe tube this close to the tympanic membrane may cause considerable discomfort for the patient. Thus, probe microphone measures may not be able to be conducted. In those cases aided sound field measures can be used to verify audibility of soft sounds.

Another important aspect of the fitting and follow-up process with any hearing aid fitting is validation of outcome. Like all hearing aid fittings, validating the results can be completed using self-reports (questionnaires). Very few published studies have compared outcomes of deep canal products relative to other instruments. Arbogast and Whichard (2009) administered the Abbreviated Profile of Hearing Aid Benefit (APHAB) on 18 users of an extended wear deep canal device. All four subscales of the APHAB showed significant aided benefit across all four subscales of the APHAB for all 17 participants. Mean benefit ratings one month post fitting of the extended wear device are shown in Figure 7–12. In addition to the subjective benefit from the APHAB scales, the authors of this study measured overall patient satisfaction across five dimensions on a 1 to 5 Likert scale, which showed patients derived high satisfaction scores with their extended wear devices. Results of the Arbogast and Whichard (2009) study support the real-world effectiveness of deep canal extended wear for the properly selected candidate. More real world studies of deep canal fitting effectiveness are warranted.

Deep Canal Fitting Checklist

Because deep canal fittings have some inherent risk factors associated with their use, a selection and fitting checklist is included to review the details of a deep canal fitting with each patient.

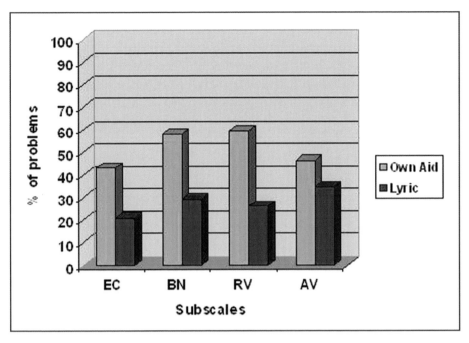

Figure 7–12. *Mean APHAB scores for the unaided and deep canal fitting condition from Arbogast and Whichard, 2009. Provided by inSound Medical, Inc. Reprinted with permission.*

During the selection process (prefitting appointment) the following issues need to be thoroughly assessed with the patient prior to fitting a deep canal device:

- Size and shape of ear canal can accommodate a deep canal device

- Cerumen and excessive moisture in the ear canal do not appear to present any chronic repair problems with the instrument

- There are no medical contraindications precluding use

- Patient is willing to give up certain features (e.g., telecoil, directional microphones) that may not fit into the small shell size of the deep canal instrument

- Patient is willing to tolerate some temporary discomfort in the ear canal related initial use

- A signed medical clearance from an otolaryngologist or medical waiver from the patient prior to the actual fitting

- The sizing and fitting protocols of deep canal products on the marketing today vary across manufacturer. Clinicians should

check with their manufacturer of choice prior to fitting deep
canal devices

■ Approximately 24 hours following the fitting of a deep canal the
patient should be telephoned so that progress and side effects
(pain, discomfort) can be monitored

■ Any changes in medical or audiologic history must be monitored
over time.

Recent Advances

Many of the cutting edge features of the peritympanic hearing aid,
introduced in the 1990s by Philips Instruments, have evolved over the
past two decades. Today, several hearing aid manufacturers now offer
mini-CIC and invisible-in-the-canal (IIC) form factors requiring a deep
microphone and receiver placement within the ear canal. Perhaps the
most exciting entrant in the deep canal fitting market is extended wear
devices. Deep canal extended wear devices can be worn continuously for
as long as four months. Unlike other deep canal instruments, extended
wear deep canal devices are placed within 4 to 5 mm of the tympanic
membrane with a special microscope. For the proper candidate extended
wear instruments are worn continuously for up to a maximum of 120
days. Therefore, these devices can be worn while sleeping and showering, batteries do not need to be replaced, and the device never has to
be repaired. Rather, extended wear instrument wearers have the device
replaced in the office by the clinician about every four months. Consequently, extended wear devices offer a different hearing aid delivery
distribution model for consumers. Instead of purchasing a single device
that is expected to last for 5 years or more, extended wear devices are
changed in the office 3 to 4 times per year using an annual subscription.
One example of an extended wear device offered to patients as an annual
subscription is Lyric from Sonova, Straifa, Switzerland.

   Considering extended wear are placed deep into the ear canal and
are not removed for up to four months, safety is a concern, as air circula-
tion is decreased to the medial portion of the ear canal for long periods of
time. Designers of the Lyric device had experience in two areas of otolaryngology that suggested an extended wear device could be placed with
minimal risk into the deeper portions of the ear canal: (1) tracheostomy
tubes (T-tubes) are placed into the tympanic membrane for long periods
of time and the surrounding tissue remains healthy, and (2) cerumen

impaction and foreign bodies can be present for long periods of times in people with severe hearing loss without affecting the health of the ear canal. Therefore, an obstruction in the ear canal, in and of itself, is not necessarily a threat to the health of the ear for the appropriate candidate.

In 2002, Insound Medical Inc. received 510(k) clearance from the American FDA for 120 days of wear and placement by otolaryngologists and in 2008 audiologists and hearing instruments specialists received the same clearance. Unlike other deep canal applications which use a customized shell, the extended wear Lyric uses in a soft and flexible seal designed to not put undue pressure on the canal wall, while still providing retention in the ear canal and an acoustic seal to minimize problems with acoustic feedback. The seals are antimicrobial and breathable and the device includes two venting mechanisms.

As the extended wear device is different from other types of deep canal devices, it's important to examine the unique aspects of extended wear fittings. Appropriate equipment is needed to visualize the ear canal. Therefore, a microscope is needed to provide excellent lighting and magnification. Otomicroscopy must be completed on all extended wear candidates prior to fitting the device. What follows is a summary of the sizing and fitting procedure for the Lyric extended wear instrument, which currently is the only extended wear device on the market. The reader is encouraged to stay abreast of other extended wear devices that arrive on the market, and be advised that their sizing and fitting procedures may differ from those reviewed here.

The extended wear Lyric can be sized and fit in by a clinician in about an hour. With proper training and equipment, the routine has been noted to be fairly simple and routine (Arbogast, 2010a). Fitting an extended wear product begins with the sizing procedure. The goals of sizing are to determine if the ear canal can accommodate the device and identify the proper seal sizes as shown in Figure 7–13.

The sizing process consists of two steps. First, a length sizer, which is a thin tube with a soft flexible tip, is inserted into the ear canal until the soft "noodle-like" tip touches the TM. Because the tip is soft and flexible, there is no pain associated with this procedure. Second, the lateral seal size is determined by using a sizer. The lateral sizer is placed at the appropriate insertion depth using slider forceps designed for placing the device at the proper depth. The quality of the fit around the circumference of the ear canal is assessed. The presence of gaps indicates the need for a larger size, whereas a tight fit and/or folds bunching in the seal indicates the need for a smaller size (Arbogast, 2010a).

After the proper seal has been indentified, the ear canal is lubricated and the device is slowly inserted to the appropriate insertion depth

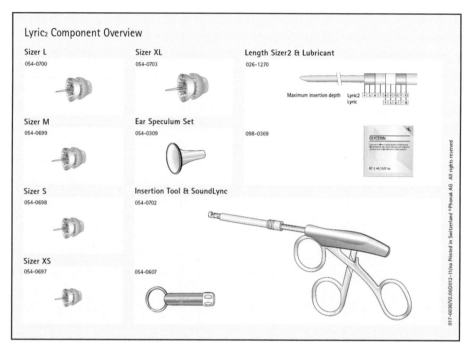

Figure 7–13. *Illustrations of the sizing tools used to fit the Lyric instrument. Provided by Lyric from Sonova, Staifa, Switzerland. Reprinted with permission.*

using the slider forceps. The clinician gauges the proper insertion depth within the ear canal based on the sizing procedure, patient feedback, and the feel of the insertion of the actual instrument to determine the best long-term placement. Once the device is properly placed it is activated with a magnet and it is programmed.

The Lyric can be removed by a clinician, patient, or another person at any time with the use of a removal tool. Once it is removed, the device must be replaced only by a trained professional. Replacement of the Lyric occurs about every 3 to 4 months. The re-fit appointment takes less than 15 minutes, at which time the patient receives a completely new device.

Given the invasive nature of an extended wear device, the health of the ear canal is a strong consideration. A group of 364 patients were studied by Scherl et al. 2011 between 2007 and 2009. A total of 64 patients (18%) discontinued use with one month due to otalgia, canal irritation, occlusion effect, or moisture accumulation medial to the device. All issues that occurred in the group of 64 patients resolved within five days and did not require treatment with a canal wick or oral antibiotics. The authors determined that the majority of these failures were the result of unfavorable ear anatomy.

In this same study, another 21 patients (6%) discontinued Lyric use after the first month, mainly due to discomfort. Other reasons for discontinuing use after one month were inadequate gain and an inability to swim. The remaining group of 279 patients was successful; however, a small percentage (9%) of them did develop some transient canal irritation associated with use, requiring the removal of the device for 3 to 14 days. All these patients were able to resume use of the device. There were no reported incidents of otitis externa, osteomyelitis, TM perforation, or sudden sensorineural hearing loss associated with the use of this extended wear device in this study. It is noted that these results are from one study from data collected from a single office, however, it does suggest that when candidates are selected and fitted properly, risk to the patient is minimal.

In addition to patient candidacy and safety requirements, deep canal extended wear devices, like the one shown in Figure 7–14, have the potential to change the economics of hearing aid delivery. Given the well-known stigma effects of hearing loss and hearing aids, deep canal extended wear devices have the potential to attract new patients, increase

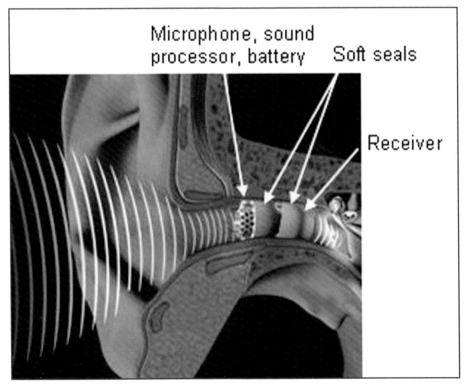

Figure 7–14. *Illustration of the deep canal Lyric device and its placement in the ear canal. Provided by Lyric from Sonova, Staifa, Switzerland. Reprinted with permission.*

referrals from current patients, and produce more revenue for a practice. A study by Arbogast (2010b) of three practices shows that approximately 75% of patients scheduling an appointment for a consultation for one extended wear device (Lyric) were new to the practices. From a business standpoint this is a favorable result, as conventional wisdom suggests that more than half of the hearing aids dispensed in a typical practice are to experienced wearers being refit by the practice. Considering how it differs from other deep canal fittings, extended wear instruments represent a disruptive technology both in terms of their device design, but also their potential to generate new revenue for a practice. Interested readers are encouraged to search for recent updates in respect to this technology as it evolving at a rapid pace.

Summary

The external ear canal plays a critical role in the successful fitting of any hearing aid. In the case of deep canal fittings, this role takes on even greater importance, as the size, shape and geometry of the ear canal affects candidacy requirements. With the recent advances of invisible-in-the-canal (van Vliet & Galster, 2010), mini-CICs, and extended wear instruments (Arbogast & Whichard, 2009), clinicians must adapt prefitting, impression taking and fitting technique in order for patients to fully realize the benefits of deep canal devices while minimizing their risks.

Considering the consumer demands of an "invisible" hearing solution, combined with the fast evolving hearing aid technology environment, readers are encouraged to stay abreast of changes by communicating with their manufacturing partners, attending educational events and monitoring credible Web sites and search engines. With the continued miniaturization of technology comes the potential to effectively meet the cosmetic and performance demands of more individuals with hearing loss. In that vein, the evolution of deep canal fittings is something to embrace.

8

Cerumen: Genetics, Anthropology, Physiology, and Pathophysiology

BOPANNA B. BALLACHANDA

Anthropologists, biochemists, dermatologists, otolaryngologists, and audiologists have all conducted numerous studies on cerumen and the secretory system. The result of one such study has been to define the material we call cerumen as a composition of secretions from modified apocrine glands, sebaceous glands, dust particles, desquamated epithelial cells, dislodged hair follicles, and foreign bodies trapped in the ear canal (Perry, 1957), whereas the secretory system consists of modified apocrine (ceruminous glands) and sebaceous glands located in the cartilaginous part of the ear canal. This chapter blends information gathered by a broad range of scientists into a cohesive account of genetics of the cerumen types, secretory gland(s), gland functions, cerumen production, and consequences of impaction.

Cerumen Types

There are two distinct forms of cerumen found in humans: dry and wet (Matsunaga, 1962). During routine ear canal examination, the distinction between these two types is quite obvious, as cerumen consistency varies from dry and brittle to sticky and moist/wet. When it is freshly secreted, cerumen has a semiliquid consistency (Matsunaga, 1962; Perry, 1957; Robinson, Hawke, & Naaiberg, 1990) that hardens with the passage of time.

The dry type (Figure 8–1) is also known as "rice bran" ear wax (from the Japanese word "Nuka-Mimi"), because it resembles just that, small, dusty granules of rice bran. It is brittle and rather flaky, and most prevalent in Asian countries, including Japan and China (Matsunaga, 1962). In contrast, the wet type (Figure 8–2) is sticky and often soft; however, a dark-hard concentration of wet cerumen is not uncommon. Robinson et al. (1990) classified wet cerumen into both hard and soft varieties: the hard type is commonly found in persons with chronic and recurrent impactions, while the soft variety, characteristically stickier and moister, is usually observed in children. In general, the wet type, unlike the dry, displays a wide range of consistency variations, from very soft to quite hard. Apart from the normal, time-dependent process of dehydration and oxidation, these variations have been largely attributed to the type of materials blended with the cerumen. For example, cerumen mixed

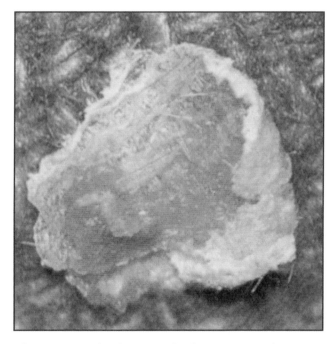

Figure 8–1. *The dry type, also known as rice-bran type cerumen. Reproduced with permission from* Diseases of the Ear: Clinical and Pathological Aspects, *by M. Hawke and A. F. Jahn. 1987, p. 2.11. Copyright 1987 Lea & Febiger.)*

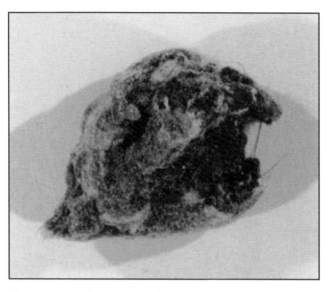

Figure 8–2. *The wet type of human cerumen. Note the hard consistency and dark color, sticky, and often soft cerumen.*

with hair follicles may appear to be harder than cerumen mixed with only dust particles.

The range of observable colors in normal cerumen is an aspect that requires special consideration. When first produced, cerumen is light to golden brown; but it has been noted that after prolonged exposure to air, oxidation and dehydration affect a gradual change in color (Matsunaga, 1962; Perry, 1957). Apart from gradual color variations, the natural color of dry cerumen is significantly different from wet cerumen. Figures 8–3 through 8–5 show variations in color; in the dry type, color ranges from light gray to brownish-gray, whereas in the wet type, color can range from brown to dark brown to almost black (Matsunaga, 1962; Perry, 1957).

Variations in the consistency and color of cerumen are related; the darker the cerumen, the harder the consistency and vice versa. Sometimes, color variations may make it difficult to distinguish cerumen from other blockages. For example, when the ear canal is blocked with a thin film of golden yellow wax, the blockage can easily be mistaken for fungal growth or another pathological condition. On the other hand, fungal growth might be mistaken for cerumen and cause one to attempt extraction. In certain cases, extracting materials other than cerumen entails the risk of creating complication that may require immediate medical assistance. It is critical that the clinician identify the color and consistency or type prior to cerumen extraction. A friendly caution about this process: soften the cerumen when it is dark and hard.

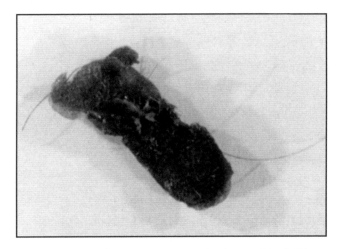

Figure 8–3. *Soft cerumen commonly observed in children.*

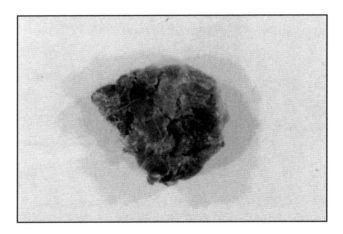

Figure 8–4. *Soft brown cerumen, keratin attached to it.*

Genetic Determinant of Cerumen Types

Type of cerumen (either dry or wet) is one of several polymorphic traits that have been discovered in humans. It is hypothesized that cerumen is controlled by a pair of autosomal alleles, G (W) and A (w), within the gene. The genotype of wet cerumen is GG (WW) or GA (Ww) and that of the dry type is AA (ww), and believed to be inherited as a simple Mendelian trait with the dry allele being recessive to the wet (Matsunaga, 1962; Petrakis, 1971; Robinson et al., 1990; Yoshiura et al., 2006). Support for this hypothesis is illustrated by a representative example of family data from Matsunaga (1962) presented in Table 8–1. The data, gathered

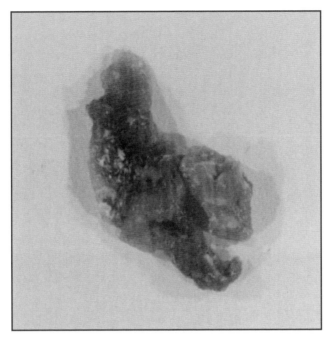

Figure 8–5. *Golden brown cerumen.*

Table 8–1. The Dimorphism in Human Normal Cerumen

Type of Cerumen in Parents	Total Number of Parents	Type of Cerumen In Children		Total Number of Children
		Dry	Wet	
Wet × Wet	14	12	35	47
Wet × Dry	116	195	205	400
Dry × Dry	191	634	0	634
Total	**321**	**841**	**240**	**1081**

Source: Modified and reproduced from Matsunaga (1962).

in Japan from 321 families with 1081 children, clearly show that cerumen type is based on single factor inheritance of dry and wet alleles.

The earwax phenotypes are inherited through two alleles at a single autosomal locus, namely, the dominant wet allele and the recessive dry allele. The frequency of the dry type are generally high in East Asian populations but are extremely rare in European and African populations. A mixed rate of dry and wet types are seen in populations from southern Asia, central Asia, and western Asia. A detailed description of the frequency of these two types of cerumen from various populations is discussed in the anthropology section.

Matsunaga (1962) was the first to identify/label the alleles for different types of cerumen. However, Tomita et al. (2002) using the linkage analysis assigned the ear wax gene locus to pericentromeric region of the chromosome16. Recent and ground breaking study by Yoshiura et al. (2006) performed genotyping case controlled study of 64 with dry and 54 individuals of Japanese ancestry using CA 134 repeat markers, as well as 54 with wet type of cerumen of Japanese ancestry using CA 134 repeat markers. They showed that a single-nucleotide polymorphism, (SNP) 538 G → A (rs7822931), in the adenosine triphosphate (ATP)-binding cassette, subfamily C11 (ABCC11) gene is responsible for the earwax phenotypes: G for the dominant (wet) allele and A for the recessive (dry) allele. The ABCC11 gene encodes the multidrug resistance-associated protein 8 that consists of 1,382 amino acids and contain 2 ATP-binding dominant and 12 transmembrane domains.

Anthropology

The genetic determinant of cerumen types in different population has been a topic of interest to several researchers including anthropologists to study the migratory patterns humans. In a discussion of an early study of cerumen type and racial differences, Matsunaga (1962) pointed out that Adachi (1937) might have been the first to uncover the relative frequencies of cerumen types among different ethnic groups in Japan, northern China, Korea, Micronesia, and Formosa. Since this early pioneering work of Adachi (1937), others have provided additional data on cerumen type in various ethnic groups. The results of these studies are compiled and summarized in Table 8–2.

It is apparent from these studies that the prevalence of cerumen types is highly variable among different ethnic groups. The dry cerumen is predominant in Mongoloid racial types found in Asia, including the Japanese, Koreans, Mongols, and Chinese. In addition, a high incidence of dry cerumen has been reported in American Indians and Eskimos (Bass & Jackson, 1977; Petrakis, 1969, 1971; Petrakis, Molohon, & Tepper, 1967). Bass and Jackson (1977) supported the Mongolian migration across the Bering Strait to North America by documenting high prevalence of the dry type in Eskimos. A finding from this study of particular importance is that the frequency of the dry type of cerumen decreased as the distance from the Bering Strait increased.

Table 8–2. Data Taken from Several Studies Showing Prevalence of Dry Type Cerumen in Various Racial Groups

Population	Sample (N)	Frequency of dry cerumen %, within parenthesis number of subjects with dry cerumen
American Indians*		
Navaho	183	63.3 (116)
Sioux	147	36.7 (54)
Nootka	244	36.4 (89)
Chilcotin	261	33.3 (87)
Aleut	140	48.6 (68)
Papago	437	59.7 (261)
Choctaw	432	20.8 (90)
Other US Indians	153	50.9 (78)
Chol Maya	81	71.6 (58)
Tzeltal Maya	68	57.3 (39)
Zinancentec	105	4.7 (11)
Mextec-Spanish	103	10.7 (11)
Cuna	90	4.4 (4)
Quechua	43	76.7 (33)
American Non-Indians*		
Caucasians	368	1.3 (5)
Blacks	51	0
Chinese	169	58.5 (99)
Eskimos in Alaska**		
Nome area	103	61.2 (63)
Bethel area	146	60.3 (88)
Wainwright	90	41.1 (37)
Anchorage	67	31.3 (21)
Aleuts, Aleutian Islands	140	48.6 (68)
Touvinians, Touva, USSR***	173	78.6 (136)
Mongolians, MPR***	74	78.4 (58)
Chinese in USSR***	281	78.3 (220)
Altaians, Mountain Altai, USSR***	190	72.6 (138)
Kirghiz of Tien-Shan and Pamir, USSR***	1277	66.6 (851)
Khakass, Khakassia, USSR***	74	63.5 (47)

continues

Table 8–2. *continued*

Population	Sample (N)	Frequency of dry cerumen %, within parenthesis number of subjects with dry cerumen
Kazakh, Kazakh, SSR, USSR***	145	60.7 (88)
Turkmen, Turkmenia, USSR***	155	54.2 (84)
Mozambicans, Mozambique***	66	53.0 (35)
Angola***	41	41.5 (17)
Russians, Frunze, USSR***	207	34.8 (72)
German[+]	514	3.10 (16)
English[+]	125	2.25 (3)
Icelandic[++]	322	1.20 (4)
Finnish[++]	323	2.50 (8)
Spanish—Basque[++]	491	5.09 (25)
Spanish—Castilian[++]	308	2.27 (7)
Spanish—Andalusian[++]	209	0.96 (2)
Greek[++]	81	6.17 (5)
Japanese population—age above 20 years[+++]	642	77 (498)
Japanese—Sapporo middle school students[+++]	1638	81 (1327)
North Chinese (Adachi, 1937)[+++]	216	96 (205)
Koreans (Adachi, 1937)[+++]	381	92 (352)
Mongols (Kinoshita, 1939)[+++]	321	91 (291)
Mongols (Imamura, 1942)[+++]	778	87 (675)

*Petrakis (1969); *Petrakis et al. (1967); **Bass & Jackson (1977); ***Ibraimov (1991); [+]Matsunaga (1962); [++]Petrakis (1971); [+++]Matsunaga (1962).

The wet type is typically seen in whites, blacks, and the populations of Africa. Surprisingly, Ibraimov (1991) reported that the people of Mozambique, Angola, and Ethiopia exhibited a high frequency of dry cerumen in contrast to the wet type observed in other parts of Africa. The reasons for this departure from the usual pattern are unknown. A combination of wet and dry types is seen in populations of certain parts of the Middle East and southeast Asia, such as Afghanistan, India, Iran, Malaysia, and Turkey (Petrakis, 1971). Given the fact that *Homo sapiens* originated from Africa and migrated to Mongolia then the gene type should have been wet type, instead the studies have indicated that they have predominantly dry type. This begs the question of what might have prompted the gene to mutate and change its behavior. A study by Ohashi, Naka, & Tsuchiya (2011) examined the possible reasons for change in ear wax type in the East Asian population compared to others. An important finding from this study clearly identified that rs17822931 had undergone a geographically restricted positive selection and changed to rs1822931—A. The reason for this change is thought to have been due to much colder living conditions of the ancestral East Asian population. Therefore, less sweating, resulting in no body odor, is considered an adaptation to extreme cold conditions. The cold conditions might have been the main trigger point, but other factors such as poor sunlight and microbial environment may have played a role.

Several factors such as selection, racial intermixture, and random genetic drift, which is of particular significance when a population of small size is isolated or has immigrated, has been attributed to the differences in the cerumen observed in various racial types. These factors have helped anthropologists to determine the migratory patterns of various races and intermixture within and between different ethnic groups. However, the discernible differences in the type of cerumen across several racial groups in the frequency of cerumen type (i.e., wet or dry) cannot be accounted for by either random genetic drift or racial intermixture alone. Could it be due to natural selection? If the type of cerumen is a natural selection, then what is its importance to humans? The selective forces that maintain this polymorphism across different racial types have not been identified. However, recent studies have attempted to determine whether an association between cerumen type and the functions of other apocrine glands exists.

Association Between Cerumen Glands, Body Odor, and Mammary Glands

From a histological point of view the cerumen gland is a kind of sweat gland or apocrine gland, like the axillary glands and mammary glands of the breast. Not only are these glands structurally similar, but they also exhibit similar physiological reactions to heat, certain drugs (e.g., acetylcholine), and mechanical reactions (Perry, 1957). As a result two important associations have been established between the cerumen type and the other apocrine glands (i.e., the axillary sweat glands and the mammary glands).

First, the axillary sweat glands were better developed in persons with the wet type rather than the dry type. Matsunaga (1962) reported that an individual's body odor was dependent on the development of axillary sweat glands, and these glands were more numerous in persons with odor than in persons without odor. Stated differently, it appears that the allele responsible for wet type cerumen also controls the growth of sweat glands which are responsible for body odor. Although the odor does not affect health, axillary osmidrosis (AO) is a condition in which the individual feels uncomfortable with his/her axillary odor, irrespective its strength, may seek medical/surgical intervention.

Matsunaga (1962) hypothesized that "in view of the association between wet cerumen and development of apocrine sweat glands or axillary odor, it may be assumed that the effect of genes responsible for earwax type is concerned with certain metabolic processes, presumably of lipid material through which individuals with different types of cerumen may display different reactions to environment" (p. 284).

Second, there is an interesting relationship between type of cerumen and prevalence of breast cancer among different populations throughout the world. Petrakis (1971) pointed out that breast cancer incidence rates varied widely in different parts of the world and were distinctly lower in Oriental countries, while intermediate in eastern Europe and the Middle East compared to western Europe and the United States. The type of cerumen also varied among these populations (i.e., dry type in Orientals, wet in western Europe and the United States, and a mixture of wet and dry in the Middle East and some parts of Asia). Petrakis and associates (Petrakis, Ernster, Sacks, et al., 1981; Petrakis, King, Lee, & Miike, 1990; Petrakis, Lowenstein, Wiencke, et al., 1993; Petrakis, Mason, Lee, et al., 1975) have since conducted several studies to determine the relationship between cerumen type and the secretory functions of the apocrine glands of the breast. Based on their studies, women with genetically determined dry cerumen, compared to women with wet cerumen, have lower metabolic and secretory activity of the breast epithelium and thus lower exposure to the potentially damaging substances that can cause breast diseases (Petrakis, 1983). The importance of cerumen type has been a topic of interest to several researchers. It is hoped that cerumen type may provide a greater understanding of an individual's predisposition to genetic or environmental factors. Even though the association between breast cancer and cerumen type is controversial (Petrakis, 1971), preliminary findings by Toyoda et al. (2009) using genotyping revealed that the allele of 538 G (Wild type) in the ABCC11 gene is associated with risk of breast cancer among a total of 416 Japanese women as compared with the 538A (dry type) allele. The SNP typing method proposed by Toyoda et al. (2009) will provide a practical tool to examine the relationship between wet type cerumen and breast cancer.

Miura et al. (2007) reported that the type of cerumen has a strong association with colostrum level. Colostrum (also known colloquially as beestings, bisnings, or first milk) is a form of milk produced by the mammary glands of mammals in late pregnancy. Most species will generate colostrum just prior to giving birth. Colostrum contains antibodies to protect the newborn against disease, as well as being lower in fat and higher in protein than ordinary milk. Miura et al. (2007) collected colostrum from 225 Japanese women who had dry (155 with AA homozygotes) and wet (70 with GA heterozygotes or GG homozygotes) cerumen. The frequency of dry-type women without colostrum secretion (105/155 or 67%) was significantly higher (p <0.0002) than that of wet-type women without colostrum secretion (28/70 or 40%). The women with the dry type seem to produce very little or no colustrum compared to women with the wet type of cerumen. Miura et al. (2007) have demonstrated that colostrum secretion from the mammary gland is associated with earwax type; however, the implication of this finding needs further research with respect to child rearing issues or an association between earwax type and prevalence of breast cancer in various populations.

Cerumen-Producing Glands

An artist's sketch of ceruminous (apocrine) and sebaceous glands is depicted in Figure 8–6. The number of ceruminous glands ranges anywhere from 1,000 to 2,000 and their distribution is mostly along the entire circumference of the cartilaginous section of the ear canal (Perry, 1957); the numbers quoted above reflect average glands for persons with wet cerumen. However, the number may be less in persons with dry cerumen since clinical observation suggests that one of the reasons for dry cerumen, in addition to the genetic factor, is the scarcity of ceruminous glands (Perry, 1957, Stoeckelhuber, Matthias, Andratschke, Stoeckelhuber, Koehler, Herzmann, Sulz, & Welschhuman, 2006). The most recent study by Stoeckelhuber et al. (2006), using light and electron microscopy, has confirmed the finding of previous researchers that is detailed under the section: anatomy of apocrine and sebaceous glands.

Anatomy of the Ceruminous-Apocrine Glands

The individual ceruminous gland is tubular and the ducts may open directly into the lumen of the hair follicle or onto the epidermal surface

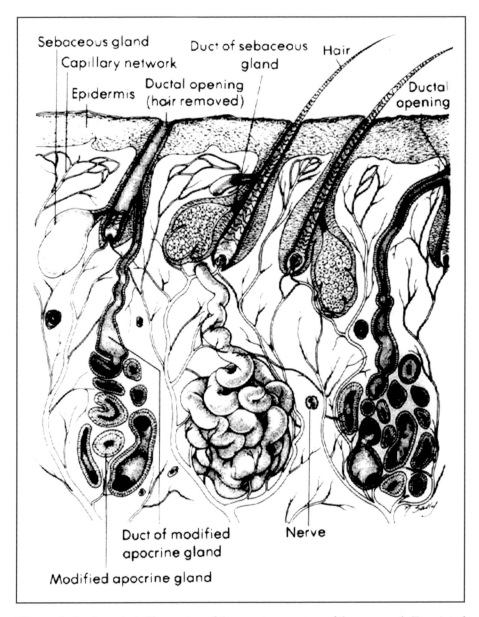

Figure 8–6. *An artist's illustration of the secretory system of the ear canal. (Reprinted with permission from "The Human External Auditory Canal Secretory System: An Ultrastructural Study" by T. Main and D. Lim, 1995, p. 1166.* Laryngoscope, 86. *Copyright 1975* Laryngoscope, 1164–1176. *Reprinted with permission.)*

of the skin. Morphologically the ceruminous glands are composed of: (1) the secretory inner sac responsible for secretion; (2) the myoepithelial outer sac, a covering that provides contractile mechanism for excretion; and (3) the ducts to convey the products to the skin layer (Main & Lim, 1976; Perry, 1957), as shown in Figures 8–6 and 8–7.

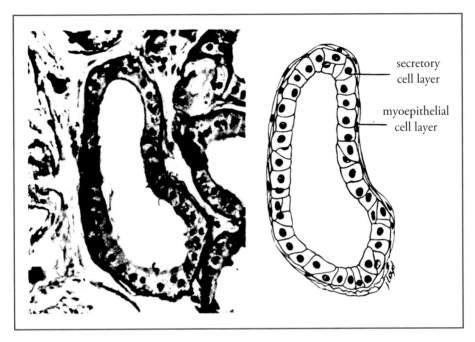

Figure 8–7. *Diagrammatic representation of cerumen gland. Note the inner secretory cell layer and the outer myoepithelial cell layer. (Reproduced with permission from* The Human Ear Canal *by E. T. Perry, 1957, p. 14. Copyright 1957. Charles C. Thomas.)*

The inner sac is lined with a single layer of secretory cells resting on the cells of the outer layer (see Figure 8–7). These cells are columnar in orientation and exhibit considerable variation in height even within the same secretory tubule. According to Main and Lim (1976) and Testa-Riva and Puxeddu (1980), the height differences may simply reflect the different stages of the secretory cycle. For example, lower or flattened cells might represent the beginning or final stages of secretory processes, whereas the tall cells might represent the last stage of the maturation, prior to secretions. This assumption holds good as the apocrine mode of secretion leads to lowering of the cell height. The secretory cells contain abundant organelles, which include mitochondria, Golgi bodies, granules (either dark/gray or light), and abundant smooth endoplasmic reticulum. These cells are endowed with microvilli, also known as buds, and the presence of these microvillus has been attributed to the maturity of the cells (i.e., the fewer the microvillus, the less active the cell) (Main & Lim, 1976). These microvilli or buds represent the part of the cell that is about to be cast off into the lumen during secretion.

There do not appear to be any morphological differences in the ceruminous glands, including the secretory cells in the inner sac, between males and females. However, there are strong indications that morphological differences exist between the secretory cells of wet and dry cerumen glands.Shugyo et al. (1988) examined the secretory cells of wet and dry type ceruminous glands in 10 subjects (4 had wet type and 6 had dry type). The majority of the differences between the secretory cells of the wet and dry types were observed in the tall cells instead of the medium or low (short) cells. The notable distinctions between the tall cells of wet and dry glands were that: (a) the Golgi apparatus was well developed and large in the wet, and well developed but considerably smaller in the dry type; (b) light granules were abundant in the cytoplasm of the wet cells, while the granules in the cells of the dry type glands were very few in number; and (c) regarding differences in the appearance of the apical protrusions, the cells of the wet type appeared large and the round processes bore "microvilli and light grains," whereas the cells of the dry type contained large protrusions, but appeared slender and lacked microvilli and granules. These differences between dry and wet cerumen glands noted by Shugyo et al. (1988) confirm earlier findings of Main and Lim (1976) and Testa-Riva and Puxeddu (1980) in persons with wet type, and the findings of Kurosumi and Kawabata (1976) in dry type glands. As a final note they suggested that the morphological differences observed in the apical protrusions (microvillus) of the wet type might account for the softer consistency in the wet cerumen.

The outer sac of the ceruminous gland is composed of smooth muscles called myoepithelium, which, by their contraction, can compress the lumen of the inner secretory sac forcing the ejection of its content. The myoepthelia cells are spindle shaped and usually appear small. These cells are arranged along the entire length of the tubular portion of the ceruminous glands up to their transition into the duct (Craigmyle, 1984; Perry, 1957). The major function of the myoepithelial outer sac is to provide a contractile function thus facilitating expulsion of the contents of the secretory inner sac into the duct.

The duct of the cerumen gland reveals two layers of poorly defined cells. It is lined by cuboidal cells similar to the secretory cells and does not contain myoepithelial cells; therefore, it may not contribute to the peristaltic contraction of the gland. These ducts usually run straight upward through the dermis and open at the middle portion of the hair follicles or on the free epidermal surface (see Figure 8–6).

Anatomy of the Sebaceous Glands

The sebaceous glands as shown in the Figure 8–6 are located closer to the skin layer compared to apocrine glands. Sebaceous glands observed in the ear canal share the same morphological and physiological characteristics with other sebaceous glands found in the skin. The distribution and size of the sebaceous glands vary greatly from one part of the skin to the other as well as among ethnic groups, age, and gender. The human sebaceous glands consist of multiple aggregates of acini that empty into the duct. The cells within the sebaceous gland undergo three stages of differentiation: (1) undifferentiated cells, (2) differentiating cells, and (3) mature cells (Montagna & Parakkal, 1974, p. 292). The undifferentiated cells usually rest on the basement membrane, and their surface is smooth and contains abundant free ribosomes (Montagna & Parakkal, 1974, p. 292). The differentiating cells start to exhibit sebum vesicles, and exhibit substantial changes within the cell body. The mature cells are often large and their surface is irregular with microvilli projecting to neighboring spaces. As the cells mature they are pushed toward the center of the glands by the undifferentiated cells on the basement membrane, which appear to show a centripetal movement of the cells. The sebaceous glands are connected to the skin by a duct of stratified epithelium.

Physiology of Cerumen Glands

Ceruminous—Apocrine Glands

Controversy exists regarding the mode of secretion of ceruminous glands; according to some investigators, the mode of secretion is apocrine (Main & Lim, 1976; Testa-Riva & Puxeddu, 1980), whereas others believe it is eccrine. According to Montagna and Parakkal (1974, p 353), "the name apocrine was given because the free end of the cell is pinched off into the lumen when the myoepithelial cells contract." The eccrine mode involves fluid secretion without removing cytoplasm from the secreting cells, this type of secretion is observed in small sweat glands present in the skin. Testa-Riva and Puxeddu (1980) identified several sequential steps during the secretory process and suggested that the mode of secretion of ceruminous glands is apocrine. Testa-Riva and Puxeddu (1980) offered the following detailed account of the secretory mechanism: "First, cellular apices bulge into the lumen forming apical protrusions. Second, secretory vesicles begin to appear at or near the base of the apical protrusion and fuse their membranes with one another and with lateral plasmalemma. Third, this continuous exocytosis constricts the base of the projection until its detachment from the cell" (p. 364).

This manner of secretion is also called the decapitation or apocrine mode. The secretory cells exhibit balloon-like enlargements that decapitate or detach themselves from the cell (Craigmyle, 1984; Testa-Riva & Puxeddu, 1980). According to Perry (1957), ceruminous glands have large lumen to serve as "reservoirs" where the secretions are produced at a constant and steady phase and stored well in advance, until such time when they are expelled out by internal (emotions) or external (drugs and mechanical) stimulation of the myoepithelial outer sac. Perry (1957) further emphasized that once the reservoir is emptied, no amount of stimulation will excrete cerumen until the reservoir is refilled with fresh secretions; the period of time required for the production of cerumen is not known.

Although the variables responsible for cerumen production are still not completely understood, much is known about the factors that control the expulsion of the gland's secretion. Perry (1957) investigated cerumen production in 150 normal healthy male volunteers by direct visualization, using magnification of the skin of the distal portion of the ear canal. He found that injecting smooth muscle stimulants, such as pitocin, into the ear canal produced secretion in 90% of the subjects. Adrenergic drugs (epinephrine and norepinephrine) were equally effective in emptying the ceruminous glands. Among natural stimulants, emotional states of anxiety, fear, and pain resulted in increased secretion. Cerumen glands also emptied their contents when they were mechanically stimulated, by rubbing or cleaning the ear canal, for example, what Perry (1957) called "mechanical milking." Vigorous chewing was also classified as a mechanical stimulation since the action causes enough distortion of the ear canal to produce the same effect.

Factors such as heat or elevation of body temperature and chlorinergic drugs did not play a significant role in stimulating the ceruminous glands (Perry, 1957). Likewise, seasonal variations or gender did not seem to be important factors in the amount of cerumen production (Cipriani, Taborelli, Gaddia, Melagrana, & Rebora, 1990).

Sebaceous Glands

Even though cerumen is a mixture of the products of ceruminous and sebaceous glands, the physiological factors that control the production of sebum from the sebaceous glands are not completely known. Unlike the ceruminous glands, which are modified apocrine glands, the secretion of the sebaceous glands are holocrine (i.e., once the secretory cells attain maturity they disintegrate to form the sebum). In contrast to the ceruminous glands, the production and flow of sebum from the sebaceous gland is continuous.

Chemical Composition of Cerumen

The published data on the chemical composition of cerumen suggest that it contains a mixture of lipids, protein-free amino acids, and several minerals. A composite list of chemicals identified by several researchers (Bortz, Wertz, & Downing, 1990; Chai & Chai, 1980; Harvey, 1989; Inaba, Chung, Kim Choi, & Kim, 1987; Okuda, Bingham, Stoney, & Hawke, 1991; Perry, 1957; Shichijo, Masuda & Takeuchi, 1979; Stoeckelhuber et al., 2006; Yassin, Mostafa, & Mowada, 1966) is given below:

1. Cerotic acid

2. Cholesterol

3. Hexose bases

4. Neurostearic acid "a bitter substance"

5. Acid $C_{17}H_{34}NO_2$

6. Substances $C_8H_{14}NO_2$

7. Argimon

8. Cystine

9. Histidine

10. Lysine

11. Protein

12. Tyrosine

13. Amino acids: leucine, isoleucine, valine, alanine, thyronine, serine, gluitamine acid, aspartic acid, glycine, amino butyric acids.

14. Fatty acids: L-elestearic, arachidic, behenic, lignoceric, stearic, cerotic, erucic, myristic, and palmitic.

In addition to lipids and the other materials mentioned above, cerumen contains copper and iron. Because of these minerals, cerumen is believed to be toxic for fungal growth. There does not appear to be any difference in the chemical composition of cerumen between males and females (Cipriani et al., 1990; Mandour et al., 1974; Perry, 1957). However, differences in the chemical makeup of wet and dry cerumen types are evident, specifically in the amount of lipids and proteins present in them. Recent studies have confirmed the earlier findings of significant differences in the chemical composition of wet and dry cerumen (Bortz, et al,, 1990; Inaba et al., 1987). The dry type was said to contain more protein and fewer lipids than the wet; specifically it contained squalene, cholesterol esters, wax esters, triacylglycerols, free fatty acids, and cholesterol. The wet type contained only squalene, triglycerides, free fatty acids, cholesterol, and several nonpolar components and lacked cholesterol esters and wax esters (Inba et al., 1987). Bortz et al. (1990) examined the lipid content in wet cerumen and identified several lipid components; he suggested that free and covalently bound lipids might contribute to the properties of cerumen.

Functions of Cerumen

There are several functions of cerumen. It lubricates the skin lining the ear canal; acts as a water repellent; and entraps dust, hair follicles, and insects. These functions are well established by several researchers including Perry (1957). The absence of cerumen can cause dryness, irritation, and itching in the ear canal. In addition, cerumen protects the tympanic membrane and the ear canal from insects, flies, bacteria, and fungus.

Based on several studies conducted before 1957 and his own observations, Perry suggested that the primary protective function of cerumen is repelling insects. However, Perry (1957, p. 65) questioned the repellent function of cerumen based on a study which tested cerumen for insect repellent action and found that flies behaved as if they were approaching a neutral material. Instead of serving as a repellent, he proposed that cerumen protects the ear canal from insects by acting as a type of "flypaper."

Some have suggested that since cerumen contains rich nutrients such as amino acids, it could support luxuriant bacterial and fungal growth (Perry & Nicholas, 1956; Singer, Freeman, Hoffert, Keys, Mitchell, & Hardy, 1952). In contrast, several recent studies have credited cerumen for bactericidal and antifungal properties (Chai & Chai, 1980; Megarry, Pett, Scarlet, Teh, Zeigler, & Canter, 1988; Stone & Fulgham, 1984; Storrs, 1981).

To ascertain the potential antibacterial activity of cerumen, Chai and Chai (1980) suspended the dry type of cerumen against 10 strains of bacteria commonly observed in humans. The most notable effect was against two strains of *H. influenzae*: type b, the leading cause of meningitis in infants and children, and noncapsular *H. influenzae* which causes middle ear infections. How cerumen would perform on these strains in a natural situation (i.e., inside the ear canal) still needs to be investigated, since this was a laboratory investigation. In spite of these reservations about cerumen activity in the ear canal, Chai and Chai (1980) were convinced that it has strong antibacterial properties. Chai and Chai (1980) concluded that one possible explanation for the discrepancy between the bactericidal action of cerumen reported by previous investigators and their own findings may be due to the type of cerumen used for investigation (dry in this study and wet in others). This explanation is questionable since dry and wet cerumen have similar chemicals, except for lipid and protein concentration. Another possibility is related to the method of homogenization used in the Chai and Chai (1980) study. In another study Stone and Fulghum (1984) reported that wet cerumen reduced bacterial activity by 17 to 99% in several bacterial cultures. The chemical substance in cerumen that was most effective in inhibiting the fungal and bacterial growth was the fatty acid; it has been suggested that polyunsaturated fatty acids have better bactericidal and fungicidal properties than unsaturated fatty acids. In addition to well-established bactericidal activity, a study by Megarry et al. (1988) suggested that human cerumen has a significant mycocidal effect to restrict the growth of fungus.

It is also interesting to note from several studies that cerumen is absent in patients with external otitis (Hyslop, 1971; Osborne & Baty, 1990; Perry, 1957; Schwartz, Rodriguez, McAveney, & Grundfast, 1983; Senturia, 1981), which suggests that the host defense is not present when the ear canal is infected with bacteria and fungus. As an effective remedy for recurrent chronic seborrhea dermatitis, Storrs (1981) recommended cerumen mixed with glycerin as a topical application to his patients to overcome the skin problem. This may indicate that cerumen has a protective mechanism from bacterial and fungal infection. However, much controversy still exists regarding the function of cerumen in the literature, since it contains both nutrients that permit bacterial and fungal growth, and antimicrobial-antifungal agents such as lysozyme, immunoglobulin, and fatty acids.

Pathophysiology of Cerumen

Cerumen production and extrusion go uninterrupted in many individuals. The mechanism of extrusion takes place as a process of epithelial cell migration from deeper parts of the canal. This migration process is unique to ear canal skin (Johnson & Hawke, 1988), possibly due to the fact that the skin lining the ear canal is enclosed and not subjected to the usual surface contact that normally removes the dead skin layer from other skin surfaces. This migratory process is necessary to rid the ear canal from an accumulation of skin debris. Alberti (1964) gave a detailed account of the patterns and rate of migration. He reported two common patterns of migration, as depicted in Figures 8–8A and 8–8B: in

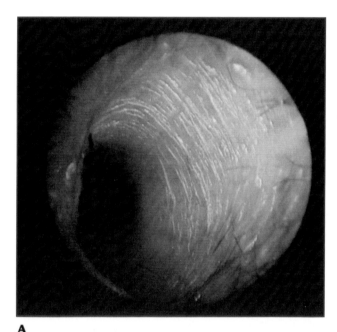

A

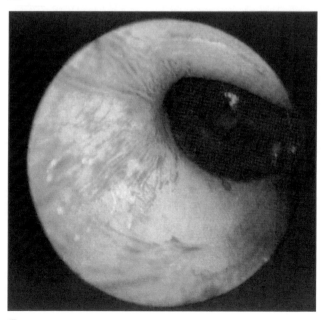

B

Figure 8–8. The migratory patterns of the epithelial layers of the tympanic membrane and the bony part of the ear canal. *A.* Radial pattern. *B.* Horizontal pattern. (Reproduced with permission from Hawke and Jahn. Diseases of the Ear. *Gower Medical Publishing, New York, NY.)*

the majority of cases (80%), it is radial away from the umbo (see Figure 8–8A); in the other cases, it is horizontal away from the handle of the malleus observed at the superior part of the eardrum (see Figure 8–8B). The mean rate of migration is 0.07 mm/day. The actual mechanism of this migration is still not completely understood; It is hypothesized that the deeper parts of the epidermis start migrating outward, detach themselves, and the desquamated material is then shed out of the ear canal by certain mechanical activities such as chewing or other movements (Johnson & Hawke, 1988).

The purpose of migration is to keep the ear canal clean and extrude cerumen out. To facilitate this process, the keratin (desquamated epithelia) has to be separated, and any disruption in the process of keratinocyte separation can cause impaction. Robinson et al. (1990) investigated cerumen collected from impacted ears in order to determine the reasons for accumulation within the ear canal. Based on histological findings and the large sheets of keratin found in cerumen, they proposed that "cerumen impaction is the result of a failure in the breakup or separation of the individual keratinocytes which normally occurs in the superficial external auditory canal. At the present time little is known about the mechanism whereby the continuously desquamating layer of deep canal stratum corneum is broken up and spontaneously expelled from the superficial external canal" (Robinson et al., 1990, p. 89). They added that the chemical compound that facilitates this detachment is not known and called it keratinocyte attachment destroying substance (KADS).

Another reason for impaction may be excessive production of cerumen due to the increased activity of cerumen glands. Mandoor et al. (1974) examined the activities of cerumen glands in persons across age and gender with and without impaction. They contended that based on histological and histochemical analyses, the glands appeared morphologically similar between the two groups, except for a marked increase in the enzymatic activities of the ceruminous glands in patients with cerumen impaction, resulting in excessive production and subsequent accumulation.

Factors such as reduction in the number of active cerumen glands combined with thicker and longer hair follicles can induce cerumen impaction in older adults (Ruby, 1986). The hair in the ear canal (especially in males) becomes thicker and longer with age, and are oriented upward and inward (toward the tympanic membrane). The orientation of hair in normal young adults is outward (toward the opening), which prevents insects from entering the canal and assists in the migration of epithelial layers toward the canal opening. Changes in orientation, thickness, or height of hair can impede this normal process and prove counterproductive for the migration of the epithelial cells and the cerumen from the ear canal. In older adults the orientation of hair follicles presents a physical obstruction and the reduction in the number of active glands produces drier and less viscous cerumen. The combination of these factors results in entrapment of cerumen in the canal and thus a higher frequency of impaction.

In addition to the above mentioned physiological variations, physical obstruction due to hearing aids, use of cotton-tipped buds, and abnormalities in the shape and size of the ear canal are also believed to induce cerumen impaction. In many cases, frequent use of cotton-tipped swabs (CTSs) pushes the cerumen into deeper parts of the canal thus causing impaction rather than cleaning the ear canal (Johnson & Hawke, 1988). Conflicting reports exist regarding the use of CTSs and cerumen accumulation. Sim (1988) and Robinson et al. (1990) argued that using CTSs did not increase the possibility of cerumen accumulation compared to non users of CTSs. In contrast, Baxter (1983) and Macknin, Talo, and Medendorp (1994) reported significant differences in the percentage of patients with impaction between CTS users and nonusers. It appears that cleaning ear canals with CTS may not produce an ear canal free of cerumen, but may increase the possibility of damaging the ear canal; therefore, CTS use should be considered potentially dangerous and discouraged (Warwick-Brown, 1986).

The amount of cerumen impaction may be partial or complete; by general consensus, complete impaction is defined as total blockage of the ear canal where the presence of cerumen makes it impossible to visualize the tympanic membrane during an ear canal examination. On the other hand, partial impaction refers to limited visualization to just half or a quadrant of the tympanic membrane, permitted by a narrow opening in the ear canal. Currently, there is no standard classification system; most studies have described cerumen impaction based on the visibility of the tympanic membrane. However, recently Crandell and Roeser (1993) suggested audiometric findings (i.e., the amount of conductive loss) as an indicator to express the amount of ear canal blockage. Their scheme consisted of three categories; *nonoccluded*-cerumen accumulation less than 50%, *excessive*-cerumen occlusion between 50 to 80% with no noticeable conductive loss (<10 dB air/bone gap at 2 frequencies), and *impacted*-cerumen impaction greater than 80%, associated with conductive hearing loss and greater than 10 dB of air/bone gap at two or more frequencies. They cited the study by Chandler (1964) to imply that conductive loss did not occur until at least 80% of the ear canal was occluded. Although this scheme appears reasonable, certain methodological factors limit such an interpretation. First, Chandler used impression materials to occlude the ear canal to determine hearing loss; the consistency between cerumen and impression material is different therefore the amount of conductive loss may be different for cerumen impaction. Second, conductive loss is not a good indicator of amount of blockage, because a small opening in the impaction can permit sound to travel to the tympanic membrane and produce no hearing loss. An optimal method to quantify the extent of blockage is to calculate the amount of cerumen by measuring the ear canal volume with and without impaction. This can be accomplished with most immittance meters.

Cerumen Impaction: Prevalence

Although cerumen impaction is common in patients seen by audiologists, there is no data exists on the actual number or percentages of patients with cerumen impaction. Berzon (1983) reported that cerumen impaction is among the most common ear problems presented in clinics of general practitioners. Reports from several studies on the prevalence of cerumen in the elderly, school-age children (Brico, 1985; Roche, Siervogel, & Himes 1978), and individuals with mental retardation (Brister, Fullwood, Ripp & Blodgett, 1986; Crandell & Roeser, 1993; Dahle & McCollister, 1986) are shown in Table 8–3. However, there is very little information on the prevalence of cerumen impaction in the general population.

Table 8–3. Prevalence of Cerumen Impaction from Different Investigators

Investigators	Number of Subjects	Prevalence
Bricco	349	10%
Brister et al. (1986)	88	22%
Crandell and Roeser (1993)	121	25%
Gleitman et al. (1992)	892	25%
Mahoney (1987)	242	34%
Mahoney (1993)	104	25%
Roche et al. (1978)	224	10%

Gleitman, Ballachanda, and Goldstein (1992) examined 892 non-institutionalized adults aged 23 to 89 years for cerumen and other audiological problems. Among the 892 subjects, 211 were identified as having impacted cerumen in one or both ears during routine ear canal examination. The prevalence of cerumen impaction in the general adult population according to age group is shown in Table 8–4.

It is evident from Gleitman et al. (1992) study that the prevalence of cerumen impaction increased with age. Gleitman et al. (1992) contended that the incidence might be higher if partial occlusions had also been included in the study.

Roche et al. (1978) found partial to complete occlusion in around 10% of a sample of children. Brico (1985) reported a high correlation between cerumen impaction and middle ear pathology in school-age children.

In the geriatric population, 65 years and older, the incidence of cerumen impaction is as high as 34% (Ruby, 1986; Lewis-Cullinan & Janken, 1990; Mahoney, 1987). Additionally, Lewis-Cullinan and Janken (1990) reported the incidence of cerumen impaction among the older population to be around 19.0% bilaterally and 15.0% unilaterally. A report by Mahoney (1993) suggested that a considerably higher number of older adults suffer from hearing loss due to impacted cerumen. From 104 randomly selected subjects over the age of 65 who participated in her study, impacted cerumen was noted in 26 subjects (25%). Of the 104 elderly subjects 21 (20%) had impaction in one ear, and 5 (4.8%) in both ears. The cerumen impaction was defined as complete occlusion of the canal with no visualization of the tympanic membrane (Mahoney, 1987). If partial impaction had been included, then the percentage would have been as high as 42% in the study.

Table 8–4. The Percentages of Persons with Cerumen Impaction Calculated According to Age Group

Age Range of Subjects (Years)	Percentage of Persons with Impaction (%)
26–44	5
45–54	15
55–64	25
65–75	34
75–84	22

Source: From Gleitman, Ballachanda, & Goldstein, 1992.

Studies have indicated that subjects with mental retardation have a higher prevalence of cerumen impaction than normal regardless of age (Brister et al., 1986; Crandell & Roeser, 1993; Dahle & McCollister, 1986). Brister et al. (1986) reported that 24% of their mentally retarded subjects exhibited excessive cerumen collection compared to normal subjects. Similar findings were reported by Crandell and Roeser (1993) from 117 adults with mental retardation. Dahle and McCollister (1986) compared children with Down's syndrome and other children with mental retardation matched for chronological age and IQ. The children with Down syndrome had significantly higher prevalence of cerumen accumulation and hearing loss compared to other groups.

The reason for higher prevalence and pathophysiology of cerumen impaction in children with mental retardation is speculative at best. A possible explanation for the greater propensity of impaction in children with Down syndrome may be due to anatomical differences in the ear canal such as stenosis, a condition well documented in the literature (Northern & Downs, 1991), and reduced diameter of the ear canal might result in mechanical blockage. Another explanation is that poor general hygienic conditions might cause buildup of debris within the canal leading to cerumen impaction.

Consequences of Cerumen Impaction

Consequences of cerumen impaction can be divided into two major areas: medical and audiological. The medical sequelae of cerumen impaction include tinnitus, fullness in the ear, pain, sudden onset of hearing loss, vertigo, and external otitis (Brico, 1985; DeWesee & Saunders, 1973). In some patients chronic coughing has been attributed to cerumen impaction (Raman 1986). In most instances the prevailing symptoms are temporary and once the cerumen is removed, several of the problems experienced by the patient disappear or cease to exist.

The common outcome of a gradual cerumen buildup in the ear canal is a sudden hearing loss noticed by the patient most often in the morning or just after showering. The type of loss is usually conductive unless the patient has had a history of sensorineural loss. The hearing returns to normal or to the level prior to impaction after successful removal of the cerumen and no further problems are observed until another episode of cerumen impaction and sudden hearing loss after several days or years. Most of the symptoms experienced by these patients can be attributed to the ear canal blockage, which not only causes conductive loss but also exerts pressure on the neural and vascular systems in the canal.

Ear canal impacted with cerumen is the major obstacle for physicians to evaluate the status of middle ear conditions, such as otitis media (Schwartz, Rodriguez, McAveney, & Grundfast, 1983). In all cases clearing the ear canal obstruction is imperative to diagnosing a middle ear problem. Schwartz et al. (1983) suggested that a common belief among several physicians is that the heat produced by the middle ear condition would dissolve the cerumen, and therefore, the presence of cerumen would exclude the possibility of any middle ear problem. Contrary to this notion, Schwartz et al. (1983) reported that cerumen was removed in 89 (29%) of the 279 children aged 2 to 60 months in whom they had identified and diagnosed acute otitis media. The younger the children, the greater the prevalence of cerumen accumulation which inhibited ear canal examination (e.g., in infants aged 2 and 12 months, cerumen was removed in 35 of the 61 (57%) children to arrive at a diagnosis). Thus, lack of visualization may very well obscure a middle ear problem and the condition may go undetected in many children for a very long period. Due to the development and introduction of infrared thermometers, the medical community has shown substantial interest in considering the ear canal thermometer as a viable alternative to oral and rectal readings. Among the several concerns, the primary one is the effect of impacted cerumen on the temperature readings. Also, the problem could occur if the thermometer pushed the cerumen deeper into the canal. Cerumen impaction appears to be a problem only if the ear canal is completely blocked.

Audiological Concerns

Impacted cerumen in the ear canal is a common finding in patients seen by audiologists. Until recently, audiologists contended that, as long as there was an opening for the sound to travel through, the test results would not be affected by ear canal obstructions (Ballachanda, 1993). However, most practitioners now believe that cerumen impaction adversely affects the audiological test results and restricts them from performing most of the tests in the audiological battery including: otoacoustic emissions, real-ear hearing aid measurements, electrocochleography (ECochG), electronystagmography (ENG), and immittance measures as well as other more traditional tests. A complete blockage can restrict audiologists or others interested in evaluating auditory capabilities from performing simple tests such as pure-tone (air and bone conduction) and speech audiometry.

Although partial impaction permits restricted view of the tympanic membrane, tests such as ECochG, ABR, and OAE cannot be performed for two reasons: (1) it is difficult to reduce the skin resistance with cerumen impaction, which can alter the morphology of the waveforms recorded; and (2) the presence of cerumen undoubtedly will change the resonance characteristics of the ear canal, thus altering the acoustic properties of the sound reaching the tympanic membrane. In addition, the accumulation can clog the probe tube, thus attenuating the level of the sound.

It is important to understand that regardless of the reasons for higher prevalence of cerumen accumulation, the impacted cerumen invariably causes conductive hearing loss which can substantially hinder psychoeducational and psychosocial development, particularly for intellectually challenged children and older adults. Myers, Siegfried, and Pueschel (1987) reported a case of pseudodementia (social unresponsiveness, impaired receptive and expressive language skills, and extremely limited verbal comprehension) due to cerumen impaction in a 16.5-year-old girl who was mentally retarded. The condition was reversed to the previous levels of functioning immediately after cerumen removal. This case study demonstrated that decreased hearing due to cerumen impaction should not be overlooked in intellectually challenged individuals, and periodic physical examinations should include ear canal inspection to avoid cerumen-related hearing loss.

Conductive loss due to cerumen impaction is frequently an overlooked condition among elderly adults. The prevalence of cerumen impaction is also considerably higher (anywhere between 25 to 35%) in individuals who are 65 years and older. Some elderly individuals may not realize that their hearing might be reduced due to cerumen impaction and thus not seek treatment. Regrettably, several audiologists and physicians do not think cerumen is a factor for hearing loss in older adults, because the hearing impairment observed in this population is most often interpreted to be due to presbycusis only and not due to any other causes. It is important that treatable causes, such as cerumen impaction be identified to mitigate any hearing related problems that might have serious consequences toward the functional, social, and emotional adjustments in older adults.

A significant number of hearing-impaired persons use hearing aids to overcome the difficulties imposed by hearing loss. The common types of hearing aids currently available to a hearing impaired persons are: (1) behind the ear (BTE), (2) in the ear (ITE), (3) in the canal (ITC), and (4) completely in the canal (CIC). With the exception of the BTE hearing aids, which uses an earmold to deliver the sound, all the other types of aids reside inside the ear canal. The cerumen is produced in the ear canal and as it migrates toward the entrance of the canal, foreign bodies such as dirt, dust and other small particles adhere to it and are extruded with the cerumen as it is cast off from the canal (Roeser, 1997). This "conveyor belt" process as in studies by Albert (1964) has shown this as an ongoing process in most individuals. Normal cleansing of the ear canal occurs as a result of epithelial migration and the action of the jaw during chewing and talking. However, the normal migratory process can be disturbed by the presence of objects such as hearing aids or ear plugs used in hearing protection devices (Ballachanda, 1995; Roeser, 1997). Perry (1956) suggested that the presence of a foreign object can result in stimulation of cerumen producing glands leading to excessive production and he termed this process "mechanical milking." It is apparent from clinical observation in patients with hearing aids that they have higher propensity for cerumen impaction.

Patients who use hearing aids are faced with several problems due to cerumen impaction: (1) Irrespective of the type of hearing aids being used, any time the ear canal is impacted with cerumen it can cause changes in the resonance properties of the canal leading to differences in the sound quality being perceived by the patient (Ballachanda, 1997). A significant problem for hearing aid users, especially for those hearing aids where the speaker resides in the canal, is the damage caused by cerumen. (2) Cerumen accounts for 70 to 80% of hearing instrument failures. Every time an ITE instrument is inserted in the ear, there is the possibility of wax entering the vent or receiver. The ear-worn instrument receiver may also become saturated with cerumen over time as a result of the vaporization and capillary action of liquid cerumen (Figure 8–9). The receiver itself is electrically charged, drawing atomized cerumen into all areas of the receiver by the charged, sound-generating coil. The receiver acts further as a heat sink. During the heating cycle caused by the warm ear and the heat generated due to electrical operation, it is likely that a "creep factor" causes the wax to flow into the receiver (Figure 8–10). The cooling cycle, which occurs during the "off" mode, facilitates congealing liquid cerumen in the receiver. The resulting added mass of cerumen on the receiver diaphragm causes low-output distortion and loss of high-frequency response. A more insidious process occurs as the acidic compounds within the cerumen slowly deteriorate the diaphragm suspension, resulting in receiver failure.

The most reported problems are listed below:

1. Hearing aid feeds back

2. Hearing aid is not loud enough

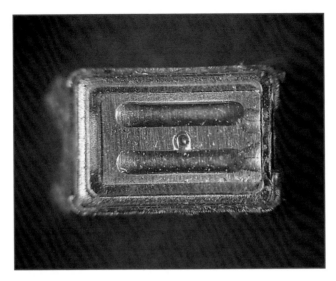

Figure 8–9. *Microscopic top view of new receiver diaphragm. E. Desporte, R. Juneau, and G. Sigele of General Hearing Instruments, New Orleans.*

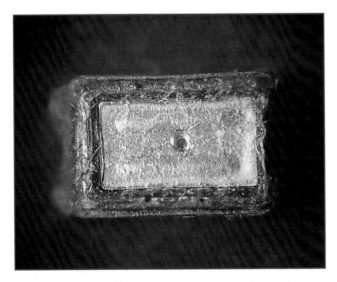

Figure 8–10. *Microscopic top view of deteriorated receiver diaphragm suspension that has been invaded by cerumen. E. Desporte, R. Juneau, and G. Sigele of General Hearing Instruments, New Orleans.*

3. Hearing aid receiver is clogged with cerumen

4. Hearing aid receiver is not working

5. Corrosion of hearing aid receiver.

In order to prevent patient hearing loss due to hearing aid deterioration, consider the following protocols:

■ Documenting improved outcomes after cleaning

■ Cost of hearing aid repair

■ Well-care visit is an opportunity to assess and prevent (as are other visits)

■ Describe appropriate physical examination

■ Choice of treatment—damage to hearing aid/loss of hearing aid in nursing homes

■ When to replace the HA after treatment?

Summary

Review of the secretory mechanisms of the ear canal indicates that the secretions of the ceruminous/apocrine and sebaceous glands are responsible for the production of cerumen in the ear canal. Among several polymorphic traits noted in humans, the type of cerumen either (wet or dry) is genetically determined. As a result, dimorphism of cerumen has been extensively studied by anthropologists and others to determine the racial intermixture and migratory patterns of various racial groups, as well as the relationship between secretions of other apocrine glands such as the sweat glands and mammary glands. Recently, hearing health professionals are becoming increasingly concerned about cerumen impaction and its consequences on audiological findings. As hearing care providers, our responsibility includes the management of patients with cerumen impaction. Cerumen management involves both identification and extraction. This chapter has addressed several issues related to cerumen, with the hope that hearing health professionals and others will appreciate and benefit from the knowledge that has been gathered by several researchers in this area.

9

Cerumen Management

BOPANNA B. BALLACHANDA

Introduction

Much of the discussion in this chapter relates to the topic of managing patients with cerumen impaction. The previous chapter on cerumen (Chapter 8) described the various types of cerumen, prevalence of cerumen impaction and consequences of cerumen impaction on audiological services. Cerumen impaction is perhaps the condition most frequently observed by audiologists during a patient's ear canal examination. Approximately 2 to 6% of the general population in the United Kingdom suffers from cerumen impaction at any given time (Guest, Greener, Robinson, et al., 2004). Four percent of primary care patients will consult their clinician for cerumen impaction, and cerumen removal is the most common ear, nose, and throat procedure performed in the primary care setting in the United Kingdom. Applying these rates to the United States population suggests a prevalence of cerumen impaction of 12 million individuals, ranging between six and 18 million. Furthermore, approximately eight million ear irrigations are performed annually for this condition (Grosan, 1998).

Audiologists have several treatment choices to manage cerumen impaction, including observation; use of cerumenolytic agents; irrigating the ear canal; or manual removal using suctioning and instruments. Combinations of these treatment options can also be used to optimize the removal process (e.g., cerumenolytic followed by irrigation; irrigation followed by manual removal). An important prerequisite to effective and competent cerumen management is the training, skill, and experience of the clinician; it also plays a significant role in the selection of the treatment option (Freeman, 1995). In addition, patient presentation, preference, and the urgency of the clinical situation influence choice of treatment (Roland et al., 2008).

A Comprehensive Approach to Cerumen Management

Considerable work was undertaken, in this chapter, to review the literature and provide evidence and value-based practice protocol. We hope that this chapter serves as a guideline for audiologists and hearing care practitioners to perform cerumen management. By definition, guidelines are intended to reduce inappropriate variations in clinical care, to produce optimal health outcomes for patients, and to minimize harm. Evidence-based statements reflect both the *quality of evidence* and *the balance of benefit and harm* that is anticipated when the statement is followed. On the other hand the value-based practice reflects patient perceived value by the intervention of removing earwax. For example, removal cerumen causing feedback for a patient with hearing aids not only relives hearing a high pitched sound, which can cause annoyance to others around, but it also helps the patient to hear amplified sounds better. In this case, the perceived value for the patient is more than simple removal of cerumen or cleaning of the ear canal.

A comprehensive approach includes all aspect of the clinical management of cerumen impaction; therefore, topics such as educational background, training, diagnosis, need for management, various procedures, and finally patient education have been discussed in this section.

Education and Training Requirements

Although the procedures to remove cerumen are generally safe, treatment of cerumen impaction can result in significant complications. Complications such as tympanic membrane perforation, ear canal laceration, infection of the ear, or hearing loss occur at a rate of about one in 1,000 ear irrigations (Bapat, Nia, & Bance, 2001; Bird, 2003; Sharp et al.; 1990). Applying this rate to the approximate number of ear irrigations performed in the United States estimates that 8,000 complications occur annually and likely require further medical services. Other complications that have been reported include otitis externa (sometimes secondary to external auditory canal trauma), pain, dizziness, and syncope (McCarter, Courtney, & Pollart, 2007).

Proficiency in cerumen management requires good clinical judgment and appropriate training. A well-trained and experienced clinician will minimize traumatic and inadequate extraction. There are no set educational standards to perform cerumen extraction procedures, rather most audiologists are expected to gain knowledge and skills during their educational training. The only document that describes the educational requirements, knowledge, and skill was prepared by the adhoc committee on advances in clinical practice of the American Speech-Language Hearing Association entitled, "External Auditory Canal Examination and Cerumen Management" (ASHA, 1991, 1992). Since the publication of that document, several changes have taken place in our education and training of audiologists and basic requirements to perform cerumen extraction is within the scope of most training programs.

Diagnosis of Cerumen Impaction

Although impaction implies 100% occlusion, sometimes the symptoms reported or observed by the clinician may not suggest a 100% impaction. Therefore, a practical rationale for diagnosis of impaction can be, for audiology practice: an impaction is considered when an audiological evaluation cannot be performed; cerumen obstructs the flow of sound to the tympanic membrane and/or inhibits visualization of the tympanic membrane and middle ear; cerumen prevents the patient from receiving optimal benefits from the hearing aid(s). Symptoms of cerumen impaction can include: otalgia; tinnitus; fullness in the ear; pain; cough; hearing loss; and vertigo (Guest et al., 2004; Sharp et al., 1990) (Table 9–1). The presence of these symptoms should lead the clinician to examine

Table 9–1. Symptoms of Cerumen Impaction

Otalgia	Tinnitus
Fullness in the ear	Pain
Cough	Hearing loss
Vertigo	

Source: Roland et al. (2008)

the ear canal and, if cerumen is encountered, consider the diagnosis of impacted cerumen.

Several studies have shown that partial occlusion and/or non-symptomatic impactions should be diagnosed and treated. Diagnosis of cerumen impaction is appropriate when the cerumen in the ear canal prevents needed assessment, even if the canal is only partially occluded; for example, if cerumen in the ear canal prevents visualization of all or part of the tympanic membrane. A study by (Schwartz et al., 1983) examined 279 children from ages 2 to 60 months and found that 89 children of the 279 (29%) had cerumen impaction, which once removed were diagnosed with acute otitis media. Similar findings have been reported in the literature, though sparse, which suggests cerumen removal even when it is partial. If cerumen in the ear canal would compromise auditory or vestibular testing, cerumen impaction should be diagnosed and removed. Most audiology tests cannot be performed accurately in the presence of complete or partial impaction; these tests include: audiometry; immittance testing; electrocochleography (ECochG); otoacoustic emissions (OAE); auditory brainstem responses (ABR); real-ear measurements during hearing aid fitting; and obtaining ear impressions for custom hearing aids and earmolds.

Modifying Factors

During the diagnosis of cerumen the clinician should also identify factors that can modify or contraindicate the treatment protocols, such as one or more of the following: nonintact tympanic membrane, very narrow canal, ear canal stenosis, exostoses, diabetes mellitus, immunocompromised state, or anticoagulant therapy. The management of cerumen can be influenced by several factors or anatomic abnormalities of the ear canal or tympanic membrane. Anatomic factors, either congenital or acquired, can modify the approach to treatment of cerumen impaction based on narrowing of the ear canal by either limiting visualization or increasing the likelihood of trauma. A narrow ear canal can make both irrigation and manual instrumentation difficult to perform. Narrow canals can be found in subjects with Down syndrome and other craniofacial disorders, chronic external otitis, and post trauma (including surgical). Graber (1986) suggested that irrigation is contraindicated: in children or infants because perforations are more likely in this age group; in patients with tympanostomy tubes, or perforation of the tympanic membrane; and in patients with recent middle ear surgery. Stenosis may be congenital or acquired. Congenital stenosis may involve both the lateral portion (cartilaginous) and the medial bony ear canal and can vary in severity from mild constriction of the canal (EAC) to complete atresia. Diffuse exostoses and solitary osteomas of the external auditory canal are acquired bony growths that may severely limit the size of the ear canal and may trap cerumen and keratin debris in the bony canal and prevent adequate visualization of the tympanic membrane. Exostoses are broad-based hyperostotic lesions that tend to be multiple and bilateral and are associated with a history of cold-water swimming (Sheehy, 1982). Osteomas are less common and are usually solitary, unilateral, and pedunculated (Kemink & Graham, 1982). Safe and effective irrigation is not always possible in these patients; specialized equipment and procedures may be required to safely remove cerumen in these patients without undue risk. In such cases, it would be appropriate to refer the patients to an otologist/ear-nose-throat specialist for safe and complete removal by combining the magnification from the binocular microscope with microinstrumentation.

A perforated tympanic membrane or patent tympanostomy tube limits the options available for cerumen removal; irrigation is strictly restricted. The presence of a non-intact tympanic membrane may be assessed by history and/or physical examination as well as by the shape of the tympanogram. Despite the caution not to irrigate, several articles have reported adverse reaction, depending on the solution used, resulting in infection, pain, or ototoxic hearing loss. In addition, use of irrigation in the presence of a perforated tympanic membrane could produce caloric effects resulting in vertigo. Mechanical removal of cerumen is the preferred technique when the eardrum is not intact. Irrigation with tap water has been implicated as an etiologic factor in several studies of malignant external otitis (Ford & Courteney-Harris, 1990; Rubin & Yu, 1988; Rubin et al., 1990; Zikk et al., 1991). Given the reports of malignant otitis externa in immunocompromised AIDS patients, tap water ear irrigation may pose risks for that group as well (Ress et al., 1997; Weinroth et al., 1994). Driscoll (1993) has demonstrated that the pH of diabetic cerumen is significantly higher than that in persons without diabetes, which may facilitate the growth of pathogens. Clinicians who utilize irrigation in this patient population must be especially careful to minimize trauma; consider using ear drops to acidify the ear canal post irrigation and provide close follow-up. Patients who are on anticoagulant therapy are at a higher risk for cutaneous hemorrhage or subcutaneous hematomas. Careful instrumentation is especially important if bleeding is to be avoided or minimized. Audiologists should also recognize the fact that the skin lining the ear canal is the same as skin lining other areas of the body, therefore, if a patient bleeds easily due to laceration of the hand or other parts of the body he/she will have greater propensity to bleed with a slight laceration of the ear canal skin.

The initial approach to a patient with cerumen impaction should include an assessment of these factors by taking a thorough history, physical examination, audiogram, and tympanogram or a combination of all. Failure to identify such factors may lead to suboptimal care, harm, or inappropriate interventions (Roland et al., 2008). Deciding the modifying factors or contraindications to perform cerumen extraction, requires good clinical judgment, adequate training, knowledge of the ear canal pathologies and information gathered from case history, otoscopy, and audiological evaluation.

Case History

A carefully gathered history can provide important information about a patient's medical and otological history. A good case history should include probing questions about: (1) perforations of the tympanic membrane or presence of pressure equalization (PE) tubes; (2) prior or ongoing ear infections, (3) postsurgical complications; (4) confirmation of diabetes mellitus; (5) record of cardiac-related problems; (6) episodes of dizziness and vertigo; (7) presence of infectious diseases or treatments that lead to an immunocompromised state; (8) use of anticoagulant therapy; and (9) a higher tendency to bleed with slight cut in the skin.

Physical Examination

A careful physical examination of the ear canal and pinna is an important factor before proceeding to cerumen management. Good visualization is key to safe and effective cerumen management, it can be achieved by means of several instruments; a thorough explanation of the reason for ear canal examination is provided in Chapter 5.

Audiometric and Immittance Data

According to Roeser and Roland (1992), a pre-extraction audiogram and immittance data are helpful in patients whose tympanic membrane is not visible due to partial occlusion. They suggest that the presence of conductive components in the audiogram, type B or a flat audiogram with a high compliance value (suggests large cavity), or the inability to maintain an hermetic seal are indicators of perforation of the tympanic membrane or middle ear pathology. However, it is important to make a distinction between type B or a flat tympanogram in the presence of smaller compliance value, which may be due to cerumen impaction, and type B or a flat tympanogram with high compliance value, which may be due to perforation of the tympanic membrane or middle ear pathology.

Need for Intervention

Health care professionals have published a considerable number of articles and reviews on cerumen management in recent years. A review of the plethora of articles in cerumen management places management into two categories: home remedies and professional management. By description, home remedies are cerumen management procedures that are conducted without the intervention of a qualified clinician. These include inserting commonly available or specialized objects into the ear to remove cerumen (cotton swab, ear spoon, etc.). In contrast, professional management is conducted by a qualified and trained clinician who examines, diagnoses, and chooses a therapeutic treatment for cerumen impaction.

Home Remedies

Inserting Objects for Cleaning

Use of cotton swabs is a common practice among many people to either clean the ear canal after showering or as an applicator to reduce itching and discomfort due to the presence of water in the ear canal. Several surveys identified the use of cotton tip swabs as a common method to clean the ear canal. Many people choose to use cotton tip swabs because swabs are believed to clean and reduce cerumen impaction; contrary to this belief though, the use of cotton tip swabs actually creates impaction. A study by Baxter (1983) showed a higher incidence of cerumen in children whose ears were cleaned by swabs. However, another study by Sim (1988) did not report a higher incidence of cerumen occluding the ear canal as a result of the use of cotton tip swabs. Apart from these two studies, which are descriptive, there are no empirical studies to substantiate a clear relationship between the use of cotton tip swabs and increased accumulation of cerumen in the ear canal. There are also no reports on the advantages or adverse effects of the use of common objects such as hair pins, bobby pins, or paper clips. The clinician should educate the patient about the dangers of using objects that are sharp and may cause damage to the skin and complications arising due to compromised skin lining the ear canal.

The use of an ear pick or ear spoon is not prevalent in the United States; however, ear picks are a commonly used item and are preferred for ear wax removal in East Asia. Ear picks are a type of curette used to clean the ear canal of cerumen; these are traditionally made from bamboo or precious metals such as silver or gold, and now also from stainless steel or plastic. Ear picks can be used by an individual on themselves or by another person. The person having his or her ears cleaned lies down with his or her head in the lap of the person doing the cleaning. Ear cleaning is often performed by a parent on a child or among adults (by one's husband, wife, or lover). It may also be performed by professional (nonmedical) ear cleaners on city streets in countries such as China, Japan, Vietnam, and other Asian countries. Ear cleaning using an ear pick/spoon in the hands of an inexperienced person can result in laceration of the canal skin and a punctured eardrum.

Ear Candling

Cerumen impaction is an age old problem, and ear wax removal has been practiced since the ancient Egyptians and Greeks. Historic remedies have included injecting goat urine and gall and the instillation of steam into the ear canal. Among home remedies, noteworthy of some explanation, is the use of "ear candles" to remove excessive cerumen. These candles are hollow cones made up of beeswax and cloth, about 7 to 10 inches long (Figure 9–1). It is believed that the use of candles dates back to 2500 BC, which corresponds to early Egyptian times. Due

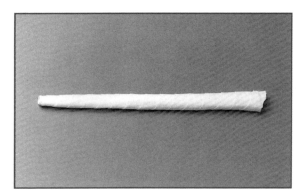

Figure 9–1. *Ear candles/ cones used for cleaning ears.*

to increased awareness of and interest in alternative and complementary medical practices, this folk remedy is now used in Europe and the United States. Ear candles can be purchased from several suppliers and it was reported that in the United Kingdom, one supplier sold one to two hundred ear candles every month, and many suppliers advertise on the internet (Rafferty et al., 2007). Proponents of ear candling claim that the candling creates a "chimney effect" thereby creating a vacuum effect that draws earwax out of the ear; the other explanation is that candling heats up the cerumen, which melts, causing liquid cerumen to come out over the days following the procedure. This extraction procedure appears to be simple and easy to perform; candling has been performed by non-medical practitioners, including beauticians, alternative therapists, or those interested in removing earwax as a home remedy. It requires few items apart from an ear candle, towel, large bulb syringe, bowl containing water and a person to assist during the extraction procedure. The person whose ear canal requires cleaning lies down on their side, the ear being candled directed upward, a pillow can be placed under the neck to hold the neck, head and back in a straight line. The candle is set at the entrance of the ear canal and adjusted to fit comfortably in the canal, if it is not properly placed smoke will go into the ear, and the process will not be very effective. As a result, care must be exercised in order to fit the candle snugly and properly in the ear canal. Following this, a towel is placed around the ear and the assistant holds the candle gently at the bottom with fingers resting on the towel. The candle is lit and allowed to burn down until it comes close to the assistant's finger, but not too close to burn. At this point, the candle can be pulled out of the canal and extinguished by dropping it into the bowl of water. The canal can be irrigated with warm water mixed with vinegar for soothing purposes and to remove any earwax left behind. The basic assumption in this procedure is that the heat (warmth) produced by the flame softens the cerumen and the pressure difference between the outside and inside of the ear canal will gently pull the cerumen out without causing any discomfort to the patient. There are no scientific data to support the effectiveness of this procedure (Rafferty et al., 2007). This is still a home remedy and, therefore, should be treated that way until new information is made available on the use of this product and procedure. Research on ear candles is limited, but several studies have reported patients suffering from burns who had no benefit from this procedure (Ernst, 2004; Rafferty et al., 2007; Zackaria & Aymat, 2009); published data do not support the claim that it can be used for ear cleaning, most importantly the use of ear candles is not supported by the FDA.

Observation of Nonimpacted and Asymptomatic Cerumen

As indicated in Chapter 8, cerumen is a naturally occurring product in the ear canal and it is extruded by normal migration of epithelium in the ear canal resulting in self-cleaning by the ear canal. If the cerumen accumulation is not symptomatic (see Table 9–1) and does not prevent visualization of the ear canal it does not always need to be removed. Patient should be educated on the importance of cerumen as a self-cleaning agent, protective function, lubrication of the skin lining the ear canal, and its bactericidal properties. Since cerumen removal is a natural process in most persons, observation can be offered as an appropriate management protocol and should not rush to remove it. Study by Crandell and Roeser (1993) reported that 50% to 80% of the residents in an intermediate care facility for the intellectually challenged were not treated for cerumen impaction but were re-examined after a year. At the follow-up examination it was found that 44% had no impaction, 53% still had some impaction and only 3% had progressed to impaction with hearing loss.

Cerumen Management by Professionals

Apart from the home remedies and non-therapeutic management mentioned above, there are several excellent papers in professional journals explaining different procedures and protocols to manage cerumen impaction effectively and safely (Ballachanda, 1992, 1993; Ballachanda & Peers, 1992; Bradley, 1986, Burgess, 1977; Carne, 1980; Graber, 1986; Larsen, 1976; Marshall & Attia, 1983; Mawson, 1974; Roeser, Adams, Roland, & Wilson, 1992; Roeser & Roland, 1992; Salomon, 1967). The type of procedure and the protocol vary from clinic to clinic. Sharp, Wilson, and Bar-Hamilton (1990), conducted a mailed survey: questioners were sent to 312 general practitioners in the otolaryngology units around the Edinburgh area to determine what methods were used for removing earwax. A total of 289 replies were received (92%); they reported that 274 (95%) practitioners preferred syringing followed by instrumentation, 12 (4%) and the remaining 5% practitioners referred their patients to outpatient clinic for removal.

It is apparent from the study conducted by Sharp et al. (1990) that cerumen management, similar to other clinical procedures, consists of benefits and risks. The risks can be minimized by identifying conditions that contraindicate cerumen extraction in some patients and by exercising precautions in others. It is felt that a comprehensive approach to cerumen management would minimize potential risks, enabling the process to be safe and effective.

Three effective therapeutic options widely used are: (1) cerumenolytic agents, (2) irrigation, and (3) manual removal other than irrigation. Combining one or more of these options, either on the same day or at intervals, is routinely used in everyday practice (Somerville, 2002). Irrigation or manual removal can be used alone or after softening the impacted cerumen. No direct comparison has been performed between same-day in-office softening followed by irrigation or disimpaction vs. home softening followed by irrigation and manual disimpaction. Until more placebo-controlled data are generated, recommendations must be based on the relative safety of the treatment strategies, on the small number of direct comparison trials within each strategy, and on expert opinion (Wilson & Lopez, 2002).

Cerumenolytics to Remove Cerumen

Cerumen that is hardened and firmly attached need not be forcibly removed. Even in the hands of a skilled practitioner, forced removal can result in laceration, injury to the skin layer, and complications. Among other things, this irritation and laceration may inhibit application of the service for which the cerumen was removed, for example, preparing an ear impression. Hard cerumen can be softened or loosened by using any of several earwax solvents. Soft cerumen may be easy to remove and less painful. Over the years several earwax solvents, also known as ceruminolytics, have been used for the purpose of softening hard and firmly attached cerumen and are also the recommended procedure to clean the ear canal. Most clinicians instruct patients to use these cerumenolytic agents at home and then remove the softened cerumen by irrigation and/or manual removal other than irrigation. All cerumenolytics come in three forms: water-based; oil-based; and non-water-, non-oil-based (Table 9–2).

Most of these products are retailed as over-the-counter remedies, principally for home use, except Cerumenex drops, which is a prescription drug. In addition to these commercially available products others agents include baby oil, mineral oil, almond oil, hydrogen peroxide, sodium bicarbonate, olive oil, and many other products used by practitioners of alternative medicine.

Table 9–2. Topical Preparations

	Preparation	Active Constituents
Water-based	Acetic Acid	Aqueous acetic acid
	Cerumenex	Triethanolamine polypeptide oleate condensate
	Colace	Docusate sodium
	Hydrogen peroxide	Hydrogen peroxide solution
	Sodium bicarbonate	Sodium bicarbonate
	Sterile saline solution	Water
Oil-based	Almond oil	Almond oil
	Arachis oil	Arachis oil
	Earex	Arachis oil, almond oil, rectified camphor oil
	Olive oil	Olive oil
	Mineral oil/liquid petrolatum	Liquid petrolatum
Non-water-, non-oil-based	Audax	Choline salicylate, glycerine
	Debrox	Carbamide peroxide (urea-hydrogen peroxide)

Source: Hand and Harvey (2004).

Therapeutic Application of Cerumenolytics

The traditional method of earwax softening or removal involves warming olive oil, sweet oil, or any other type of oil, to body temperature and pouring a tablespoon full or a small amount into the ear canal. This should soften and lubricate the cerumen, the softened and disintegrated cerumen is then pushed out of the ear canal by normal migratory process. The frequency of application of natural oils usually takes places over a period of three to four days and can range from once to twice a day.

The recommended procedure for commercially available cerumenolytics is to instill few drops (any of the commercial products in Table 9–2) in the impacted ear canal and allow 15 minutes for the drops to remain there during each application. For most of the cerumenolytics to be effective a regimen of twice a day application for 3 to 4 days would be required. In some patients, one need not go through a lengthy process of cerumen softening, instead, place a few drops of ceruminolytics into the ear canal for about 15 to 30 minutes and then irrigate with water. Cerumen removal/softening in some patients may require a lengthy period, longer than 3 to 4 days, in such instances a second visit following a regimen of softening is strongly encouraged. When softened, cerumen is easy to manage and removal may be carried out by ear curettes, forceps, suction, irrigation, or a combination of methods.

Efficacy of Cerumenolytic Agents Without Irrigation

The intent of using cerumenolytics is to either soften the wax prior to removal at the clinic or to help remove the wax on its own. Cerumenolytic agents as a single intervention have been evaluated through studies comparing active agents to: (1) another active agent, (2) plain water, (3) saline, and (4) no intervention. The reported studies are heterogeneous with a variety of treatment protocols and have used various endpoints/outcome measures to determine the efficacy of these cerumenolytic, including the need for subsequent irrigation and the ability to examine the tympanic membrane.

Kean et al. (1995) examined the effectiveness of four cerumenolytics, sodium bicarbonate and sterile water (water-based), cerumol (oil-based), and no treatment in older adults. Subjects were treated for five days prior to reassessment. They reported moderate or complete clearance of the ear canal was achieved in 32% of the patients in the control group, 50% of the patients who were cleaned by water, 46% who had used sodium bicarbonate, and 60% of the group who had used oil-based preparation, thereby reducing the need for syringing to clean the cerumen. The authors concluded that using any cerumenolytic is better than using no cerumenolytic. The finding clearly suggests that treatment with either water-based or oil-based is better than no treatment; however, the efficacy of oil-based and water-based was not significantly different. A previous study conducted by Lyndon et al. (1992) compared the non-water, non-oil based preparation (Audax) to an oil based preparation (Earex) to clear the wax without irrigating the canal. The reported findings suggest Audax was effective in 39% of the patients compared to Earex in 23%. Two other studies compared the effectiveness of different water-based preparations in both adults and children (Carr & Smith, 2001; Singer et al., 2000). Singer et al. (2000) compared the effectiveness of docusate sodium (DS) and triethnolamine polypeptide (TP); they reported that 19% of ears that were treated with DS and 9% of ears treated with TP did not need irrigation, implying that DS is more effective than TP. One systematic review and meta-analysis evaluated 15 preparations, including saline and plain water, and concluded that without syringing, there was weak evidence that both water-based and oil-based ear drops were more effective than no treatment. Non-water-, non-oil-based preparations were more effective than oil-based preparations. Pooled data from this review suggest that longer treatment results in greater success in the clearing of cerumen (Hand & Harvey, 2004).

Efficacy of Cerumenolytic Agents Followed by Irrigation/Syringing

Few studies assessed the effectiveness of cerumenolytics by measuring the amount of water or time required to irrigate the ear canal successfully following the use of cerumenolytics (Bailes et. al., 1967; Burgess, 1966; Fraser, 1970; Hinchcliffe, 1955). The conclusion of a Cochrane review by Burton (2004) of water-based and oil-based preparations concluded that no specific agent was superior to another and none were superior to either saline or water (Burton, 2004). One study of children compared a single 15-minute installation of: Cerumenex (10% triethanolamine polypeptide oleate condensate); Colace (docusate sodium), and saline drops (Meehan et al., 2002). There was no difference in the clearance of cerumen with this protocol that included irrigation if the ears were not completely clear after the 15-minute period. Children age 6 months to 5 years were treated with docusate, triethanolamine polypeptide, or saline with no statistical difference between groups after instillation of drops and following one or two attempts of irrigation (Whatley et al., 2003). The three treatment groups were similar with regard to age, sex, race, type of wax, and number of tympanic membranes partially or completely obstructed.

A strong and unequivocal finding from all these studies suggest that the use of softening agents prior to irrigation facilitated the process. However, significant differences were noted in the efficacy of various agents across these studies. Most of the studies strongly recommended using commercially available softening agents, except for one study where a 10% solution of sodium bicarbonate was markedly superior in disintegrating the cerumen in vitro preparation (Robinson & Hawke,

1989). There are differing opinions on the use of sodium bicarbonate solution (Freedman, 1990), importantly, sodium bicarbonate solution is not recommended for use in the United States.

Efficacy of Cerumenolytics in In Vitro Studies

An in vitro study of multiple aqueous solutions and organic solvents demonstrated that a 10% solution of sodium bicarbonate was the most effective preparation for disintegration of a wax plug (Robinson & Hawke, 1989). In vitro studies support using a true cerumenolytic rather than an oil-based lubricant for the disintegration of cerumen, with a longer period of treatment tending to be more efficacious. Studies that have looked into the efficacy of different cerumenolytics are not conclusive enough to recommend one product over the other, though several products claim improved wax dissolution compared to their competitors. Opinions differ as to which wax solvent is most effective and recent reports (Fraser, 1970; Robinson & Hawke, 1989) suggest that such differing opinions are strongly held, a fact which suggests that perhaps no one cerumenolytic has an outstanding advantage over any other.

Several studies have been performed to determine the efficacy of cerumenolytics and other products in clinical trials and in vitro preparations. In another study, the cerumen collected form healthy ears was placed in test tubes immersed with several commercially available cerumenolytics and other agents to study the time taken to completely disintegrate the cerumen block (Robinson & Hawke, 1989). Others have combined both the clinical trials and in vitro preparation to determine the effectiveness of these solvents in breaking up the cerumen as well as ear canal complications, such as external otitis (Fahmey & Whitefield 1982; Fraser, 1970).

Oil-based preparations are not true "cerumenolytics." They lubricate and soften cerumen without disintegrating cerumen (Robison et al, 1989). The mechanism by which non-oil-, non-water-based ear drops manage cerumen has not been defined by in vitro studies (Hand & Harvey, 2004). In summary, the evidence indicates that any type of cerumenolytic agent tends to be superior to no treatment but lacks evidence that any particular agent is superior to any other. In vitro studies support using a true cerumenolytic rather than an oil-based lubricant for disintegration of cerumen, with a longer period of treatment tending to be more efficacious.

Cerumen Extraction

Precautions

The following precautions should be considered prior to cerumen management/removal:

1. Explain the procedure to the patient and obtain informed consent to perform the procedure(s).

2. Sterilize all the instruments that come in contact with the patient, for example, specula, and other instruments. It is necessary to wash hands thoroughly before and after the procedure.

3. Use surgical gloves to avoid contact with body fluids and blood-borne pathogens.

4. Arrange medical assistance if needed in some cases.

5. Do not forcibly remove cerumen, as forced extraction may result in laceration and injury to the skin lining the ear canal.

6. Follow any guidelines set forth by the employer or regulatory board such as state licensing board.

7. Maintain a complete documentation of procedure(s) performed, and outcome of the procedures (successful removal or any complications).

Instruments for Cerumen Extraction

A large selection of instruments is available for cerumen extraction; each instrument serves a specific purpose and when used effectively, can remove cerumen efficiently and swiftly with minimal impact to the patient. In this section, the objective is to provide broad descriptions of various instruments commonly used in audiology and otolaryngology clinics for cerumen extraction, for both novice and experienced clinicians.

Curettes

Buck curettes are ideal for dislodging and retracting cerumen from the ear canal. These curettes (Figure 9–2) are available in five sizes, the higher

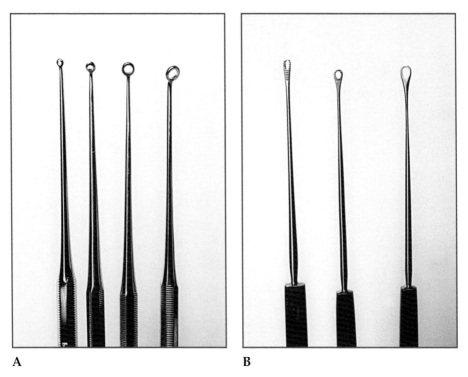

Figure 9–2. *Buck and Shapleigh ear curettes.* **A.** *Buck curettes dull four sizes (0-1-2-3).* **B.** *Shapleigh sizes (small, medium, and large).*

the number (00, 0, 1, 2, 3,), the bigger the size; they may be curved or straight. To select an appropriately sized curette for a given ear, the clinician must determine the size of the canal and the amount of blockage, it is conceivable that the larger the curette size, the greater the amount of retracted ear wax, which makes the process easy and quick. Another type, known as Shapleigh curettes, have serrated loops, available in small or large sizes for cerumen retraction.

Billeau Loops

These are similar to buck curettes (Figure 9–3), except that the loop is made of thin, stainless steel, semiflexible, malleable wires, and they come in three sizes: small, medium, and large. Loops are easily inserted, dislodging cerumen, and retracting the dislodged cerumen. The loops are strong enough to extract cerumen, but delicate and smooth enough not injure the skin lining the canal.

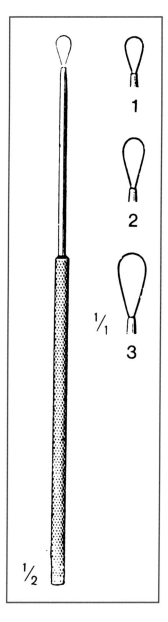

Figure 9–3. *Billeau ear loops (sizes 1, 2, and 3).*

Lucale Hooks

Hooks (Figure 9–4) are convenient to retract cerumen dislodged in the ear canal. Hooks have a blunt, round-shaped head, permitting the clinician to insert the hooks and retract cerumen without causing damage to the skin lining the ear canal.

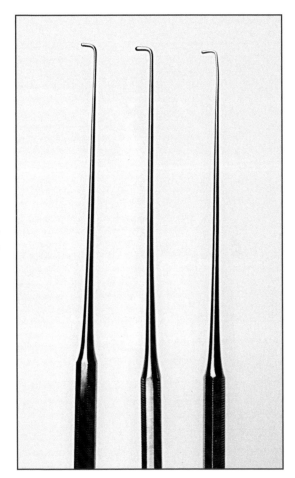

Figure 9–4. *Lucae ear hooks. Two different sizes shown.*

Aural Forceps

Aural forceps are extremely useful in removing cerumen lodged in the ear canal (Figure 9–5). From the range of forceps available, the micro-ear forceps, that is, the alligator type, among other types of aural forceps allow for greater precision to extract cerumen from the ear canal. It is small, easy to insert, and handles comfortably when in the ear canal.

Aural Suction Unit

The aural suction unit consists of an aspirator and suction tips (Figure 9–6). Aspirators can range from portable, lightweight units to powerful, multiunit suction pumps installed in hospitals or clinics. For cerumen extraction a portable suction unit will be quite adequate to

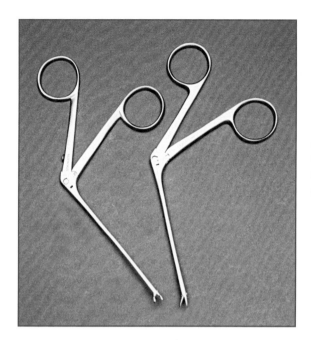

Figure 9–5. *Aural forceps: alligator and cupped. The extent of the jaw opening can vary considerably.*

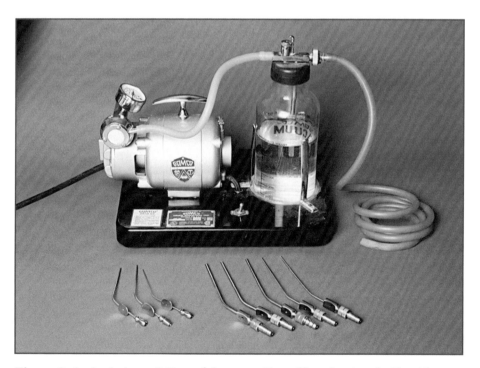

Figure 9–6. *Aspirator unit. Powerful pump with muffler, glass trap bottle with overflow protector, suction tip holder, and tubing. Placed below the aspirator unit are* Baron *(on the left) and* Ferguson-Frazier *(on the right) suction tips.*

perform the job. The factors that determine the capability of the aspirator depend on horsepower and the vacuum it creates for suctioning. A suction unit comes with a suction regulation valve and a gauge to monitor the amount of suctioning, and a bottle to collect the objects aspirated from the ear canal for disposal. Soft wax and water are best aspirated from the ear canal using suction tips. Again, there are several tip sizes, 3, 5, 7, 8, and 10. However, French sizes 3 and 5 should be adequate and suitable for most suctioning needs.

Aural/Meatal Syringe

These are metal syringes that come in a variety of sizes. The syringe has a barrel with a plunger and a conical tip-nozzle or cannulas through which the water is ejected; some syringes come with a shield to protect from back-spray (Figure 9–7). For this method, it is important to select an appropriate size syringe, otherwise depressing a plunger with a fully outstretched thumb will be awkward, and can also cause the nozzle to move unpredictably and strike the ear canal. The syringe is convenient and satisfactory for irrigation purposes. An ear basin of stainless steel or plastic is required for collecting the egress.

Aural Irrigator

Salomon (1967) introduced the oral jet irrigator as a time saving device to extract cerumen. Instead of using the apparatus in its original form, he modified the tip and added an "in-line" foot switch. The modified tip had a larger orifice to increase the flow of water, a better angle for ease of insertion into the ear canal, and the addition of an "in-line" foot switch provided better control when operating the irrigator. Using one-third pressure setting, each ear canal was cleaned at an average time of 25 to 27 seconds compared to the 6 to 7 minutes required for ear syringing.

Since the introduction of oral jet irrigators (Figure 9–8) for ear canal irrigation a number of practitioners have used it effectively and safely (Ballachanda & Peers, 1992; Roeser et al. 1992; Watkins, Moore, & Phillips, 1984). The oral jet irrigator comes with a water container; pressure pump; control to adjust the mean pressure, pulses/sec; and a tip. In addition to being faster in dislodging and cleaning the cerumen, it also provides the added advantages of controlling the water pressure, is easy to handle with one hand, and the large reservoir of water reduces the necessity of repeated refilling at short intervals. As a precautionary measure, the clinician must be made aware of the different settings for

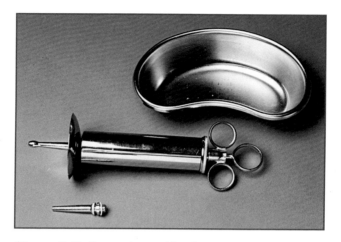

Figure 9–7. *Ear syringe with plunger, protecting shield, and cannula. Accompanying the syringe is a cannula and a stainless steel emesis basin.*

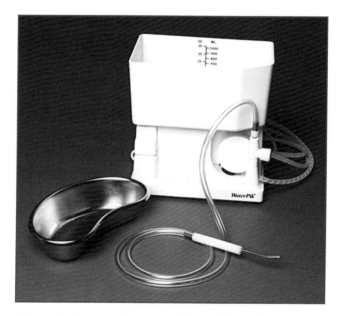

Figure 9–8. *Aural irrigator (Water Pik oral irrigator); a stainless steel emesis basin.*

adjusting the available mean pressure and pulses/sec. Not knowing these values might make the clinician prone to induce damage to the ear canal and tympanic membrane. The tympanic membrane, although resilient, is susceptible to damage under conditions of high pressure.

The relationship between the amount of pressure buildup within the ear canal needed to rupture the tympanic membrane was investigated by Keller (1958). He sealed right and left ear canals in 15 cadavers (within 24 hours after death) and increased the pressure until the tympanic membrane ruptured. The pressures required to rupture the tympanic membrane ranged from 96.5 kPa to 227 kPa with a mean pressure at 172 kPa. Interestingly, he noted that the manner in which the pressure build up took place, gradual or sudden, did not produce variations in the amount of pressure required to rupture the tympanic membrane. Therefore, it is important to remember that gradual, similar to sudden pressure build up can induce the same adverse effect on the tympanic membrane. Dinsdale et al. (1991) compared the peak pressure at full power across different oral jet irrigators and reported that the peak pressure can range anywhere from 200 to 503 kPa at the jet tip, and pulsate approximately 900 to 1200 times per minute. It appears that the peak pressure generated by these devices at full power is capable of rupturing the tympanic membrane. To avoid catastrophic damage, Dinsdale et al. (1991) recommended reducing the force of the stream either by decreasing the output pressure or by using a special tip (discussed in the next section).

The commercially available tip, that is, the tip provided with the instrument, has certain limitations: it is short, the angle of water ejection is steep, and the orifice is small hence the stream is fine. All these limitations prompted Salomon (1967) to initiate the development of a special tip. Since then, the tip has undergone changes, and the tip currently available, also known as an ear irrigator and introduced by Grossan (1978), has a couple of advantages (Figure 9–9). First, it reduces the force of water ejection, thus improving safety by directing the water stream through four jets located on the sides (Figure 9–10). Therefore, the water does not strike the tympanic membrane directly. Second, it is long, making it convenient to hold and easily direct the water.

Cerumen Extraction Procedures

Cerumen Extraction Using Instruments

To extract cerumen with a blunt ear currette, loops or forceps requires a co-operative patient who is able to remain still during the entire procedure. Instruct the patient not to move the head during extraction and to inform the clinician as soon as possible should he/she experience discomfort or pain during the procedure. Hold the instruments firmly

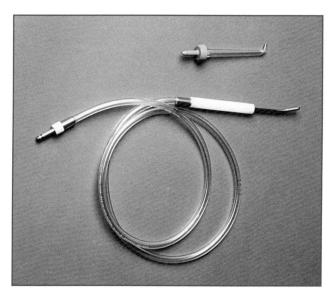

Figure 9–9. Top: *Standard tip available with the aural irrigator.* Bottom: *special tip directs the water sideways, also known as "Ear Irrigator."*

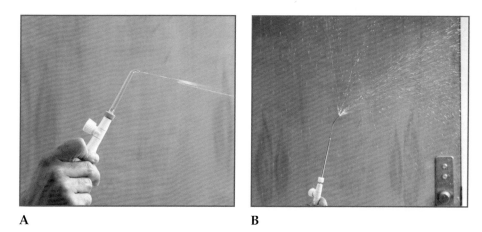

A   B

Figure 9–10. A. *The direction of water ejection in the standard tip provided with the instrument, note the flow of water, steep and narrow.* **B.** *The "Ear Irrigator" directs the water stream through flow four jets located on the sides. Sideward flow reduces the force of water ejection.*

between the thumb and forefinger, placing the hand with the instrument on the patient's head to stabilize the hand.

The safest method to perform this technique is by introducing an appropriate size currette or forceps into the canal under adequate illumination with a direct view of the canal. And then dislodge the cerumen from the epithelial layer to which it adheres and slowly retract the entire or flaked cerumen from the canal (Figures 9–11 and 9–12). If the cerumen is firmly attached to the epithelial layer and the patient is experiencing discomfort at its removal, either squirt diluted vinegar or hydrogen peroxide or place a few drops of cerumenolytics into the ear canal to soften the cerumen and render the process easy and less painful. Repeated spraying may be necessary when cerumen is hard to dislodge from the underlying skin. Care must be exercised not to remove the cerumen by force, since such extraction will undoubtedly cause laceration and damage to the skin layer. Extraction using instruments is quite effective when hard cerumen is loosely attached to the skin and clearly visible to the clinician. Attempting to remove soft cerumen using instrument may be laborious and time consuming.

After cerumen extraction, the ear canal should be inspected to confirm that the skin lining the canal is intact, there are no cuts or nicks, and the cerumen has been removed. If the cerumen does not dislodge after several attempts and the patient experiences discomfort, then the clinician should determine whether to irrigate the canal or advise further softening and a follow-up appointment after 3 to 5 days.

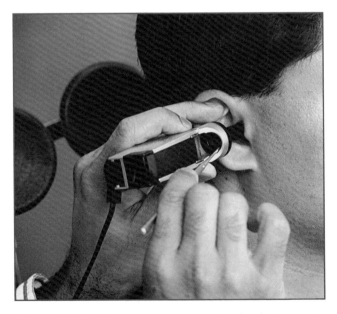

Figure 9–11. *Cerumen management using instruments. Curette being inserted into the ear canal via a Hotchkiss otoscope during cerumen extraction.*

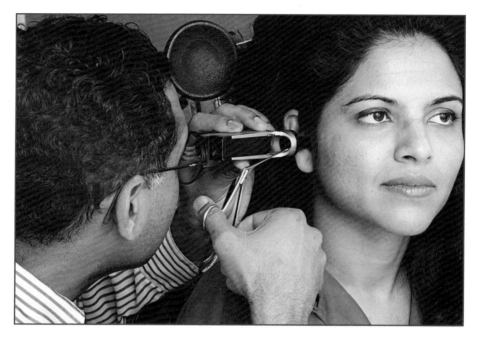

Figure 9–12. *Cerumen management using instruments. Forceps being inserted into the ear canal via a Hotchkiss otoscope during cerumen extraction.*

Aural Suctioning

Suctioning is an appropriate procedure when the cerumen is semiliquid or fragmented and has accumulated at the entrance of the ear canal (Figure 9–13). Adequate illumination and a direct view of the ear canal is essential to avoid damage to the skin underlying the cerumen. Suctioning cerumen in some cases may cause discomfort and laceration of the skin; caution should be exercised to prevent inserting the suction tip so deeply into the canal that inadvertent damage to the tympanic membrane occurs.

After suctioning, the ear canal should be inspected to ensure that the canal and eardrum are intact, and that the cerumen has been removed. If the cerumen has not been removed, then the clinician should decide whether to irrigate the canal or refer the patient to a medical facility. Furthermore, softening and a follow-up appointment should be encouraged when needed.

Aural Irrigation

An aural irrigation is not time consuming and is the most commonly used procedure to extract cerumen (Roeser et al., 1991; Sharp et al., 1990).

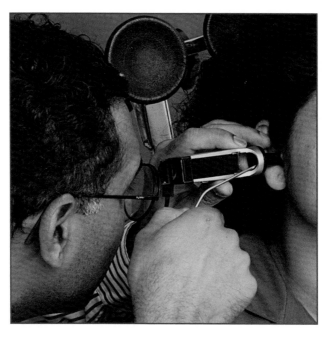

Figure 9–13. *Cerumen management using instruments. Suction tip being inserted in to the ear canal via a Hotchkiss otoscope during cerumen extraction (see text for details).*

According to Sharp et al. (1990), 95% of the physicians surveyed (total of 312 surveys) in England used syringing as a primary method to remove ear wax from the ear canal.

To irrigate the canal, either a meatal syringe or an oral jet irrigator can be used. However, the oral jet irrigator has several advantages, provided the clinician is sufficiently knowledgeable and proficient in using the oral jet irrigator. If it is used properly, it is safe and effective (Roeser & Roland, 1992). However, Dinsdale et al. (1991) reported a potential hazard of using oral jet irrigator as causing some patients to incur damage to middle ear structures, leading to loss of hearing and balance problems. They indicated that different pressure settings can cause various types of damage, and as a caution, suggested using a minimal setting. It is essential that the audiologist be aware of different settings and corresponding water pressures. It is safest to start at a low pressure and gradually increase to a comfortable and safe level.

During irrigation, water under pressure and at body temperature (37°C) is injected into the ear canal at an angle; in most instances, the water pressure dislodges the earwax, fragments it, and extrudes it from the ear canal. Irrigation has been used safely in many settings. Recently, Roeser, Adams, and Watkins (1991) have reported findings from more than 2,000 cases of irrigation without any complications. Although irrigation is a safe and fast procedure, audiologists should be aware of the risks and benefits before performing an irrigation. Graber (1986) suggested that irrigation is contraindicated:

1. in young children or infants because perforations are more likely in this age group,

2. in patients with tympanotomy tubes,

3. when the tympanic membrane is perforated, or

4. when surgery of middle ear has been recent.

   In addition, when there is a history of dizziness, diabetes mellitus, earache, drainage, external otitis, and ear canal infections, clinicians should refrain from irrigating the canal.

   The step-by-step procedure to perform aural irrigation follows.

Preparing the Patient

1. The patient should be comfortably seated in a chair, and the chair height should be adjusted to position the patient's ear canal at the plane of the clinician's eye. This ensures proper placement of the irrigator tip and direct view of the ear canal during irrigation. Once the patient is comfortably seated, place a towel over the shoulder; next inform the patient regarding the procedure(s) (informed consent) and their task during irrigation. Patients' instructions may be worded as follows:

   > Mr/Ms/ Mrs . . . I am going to irrigate your ear with warm water to remove the earwax that is blocking the ear canal. It is important that you do not move during irrigation; it is also equally important to inform me if you feel the water temperature is too cold or too warm or you experience dizziness or light headedness during the procedure. If you are uncomfortable, please let me know immediately. I would like you to hold this basin under your ear tightly pressed against the side of your face. Do you have any questions?

2. Answer any and all questions the patient might have; if there are no questions then proceed to the next stage. Tilt the patient's head slightly downward, so that the water can drain out freely.

Irrigation

1. Check the water temperature using a thermometer to confirm that the water temperature is equal to, that is, the same as the body temperature (37°C). Using water above or below this temperature can cause vertigo, transient dizziness, and in extreme cases, syncope, because of the stimulation of the auricular branch of the vagus nerve and cardiac depression (Prasad, 1984). Drain any water remaining in the tip, so that the patient will not experience sudden temperature changes.

2. Place the nozzle of the syringe or the tip of the irrigator just at the entrance of the ear canal. Care must be taken to ensure that the tip is at the entrance of the canal; it should always be visible and directed towards the roof of the canal. Proper angle can be achieved by straightening the canal—by pulling, the pinna is gently drawn backward and upward—for water delivery and ease of cerumen removal. To avoid catastrophic injuries (Dinsdale et al., 1991), set the pressure/pulses to the lowest level available and increase the pressure to a higher level only if needed. Do not direct the water at the cerumen plug this may push the cerumen deeper into the canal, instead, direct the water toward the superior wall (Figure 9–14).

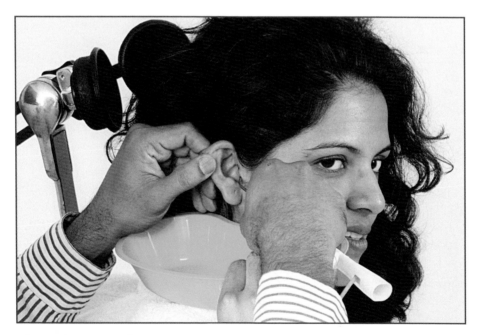

Figure 9–14. *Aural irrigation. Patient seated comfortably holding the basin, notice that the patient's head is tilted slightly downward and the ear tip is placed at the superior quadrant for the egress to flow without obstruction.*

This procedure will direct the water to sides and build pressure gently behind the cerumen plug and fragment it, forcing it out.

3. Using appropriate water pressure, direct the stream of water into the ear canal for a few moments, approximately 20 to 30 seconds (Roeser & Roland, 1992). Inspect the ear canal to evaluate the effectiveness and progress in cerumen extraction. Repeat this procedure a few more times and determine whether cerumen has been removed. Often, cerumen may be dislodged but remain in the canal, this can be removed by inserting instruments (see extraction using instruments).

4. Before removing the towel, the head should be inclined to drain any remaining water from the ear canal. Alcohol (75%) can be used to dry the ear canal. Cotton swabs may also be placed at the ear canal to absorb excess water.

5. After irrigation, the ear canal should be inspected to assure that the ear canal and ear drum are intact and the cerumen has been removed. If the cerumen has not been removed, then the clinician should decide either to extract the cerumen by instruments or suction it. Further softening and a follow-up appointment should be encouraged if needed in some patients.

Postextraction Evaluation

Postextraction evaluation involves two steps: (1) ear canal inspection, and (2) documentation of the activities in the patient's chart or file.

Ear Canal Inspection

Ear canal inspection, similar to pre-extraction procedure, is to evaluate the status of the ear canal and the tympanic membrane ensuing the extraction procedure. It is important to determine the outcome of the procedures, that is, whether cerumen has been removed completely or requires additional softening; the ear is presenting with a difficult situation that requires medical referral; or extraction procedures other than what was tried should be attempted. If referring to a medical facility is chosen then request the patient to continue using ceruminolytics, which will make the extraction process easier during the office visit. If an inadvertent trauma to the skin lining, perforation, or other complications arise, you should refer the patient to an appropriate medical facility for prompt medical attention. This requires knowing who to contact in case of emergency, and payment protocol for such medical services. One way to resolve these problems is to be familiar with insurance coverage and practice policies and privileges for the specific workplace.

Documentation

Document in detail all the activities in the patient's file or chart. An elaborate record of the extraction procedure tried; outcome of each procedure; successful extraction or partial extraction; any recommendations, and so forth. And, finally, if there is no reason for further extraction, or follow up, then proceed with audiological evaluation and other tests.

Educating Patients on Cerumen Impaction and Ear Canal Hygiene

---

Normal production and cleaning of cerumen takes places without interruption in most persons; however, this can be interrupted in few and it becomes important to educate them on ear hygine and ear cleaning. Although empirical evidence supporting measures to prevent cerumen impaction is limited, practitioners have the opportunity to counsel patients on the risks of cerumen impaction and potential benefits of ear cleaning. The population that is more susceptible to impaction are: (1) elderly, (2) persons with compromised cognitive functions, (3) abnormal morphology of the ear canal (narrow canal and anatomically abnormal canal), (4) persons who wear hearing aids and also ones who uses in the ear plugs, (5) persons with higher propensity to produce excessive cerumen, and (6) certain dermatological conditions. The clinician should counsel patients on the following issues: (1) routine ear canal checkup and cleaning by a clinician; and (2) instilling topical preparations (ceruminolytics) to keep the ear canal clean. The clinician should discuss the cost factor, treatment options, and benefits of routine cleaning. In addition, the patient should be counseled on using cotton tips, bobby pins, and other objects to clean the ear canal, using these objects can contribute to impaction or damage the structure in the canal. Patients with hearing aids should be counseled on keeping the ear canal clean, thereby hearing aid(s) damage and disruption in use can be minimized. Studies evaluating the benefits as well as the harms associated with specific interventions designed to prevent or reduce cerumen impaction are very limited, and this area of research warrants further investigation.

Summary

The cerumen management chapter has provided adequate information for audiologists who are desirous of performing cerumen management. As mentioned before, more audiologists will be involved in cerumen management in the near future. Several areas of cerumen management require attention; there is a need for standardization of procedures, protocols, and training. A well-trained and proficient audiologist can extract cerumen swiftly with minimal discomfort for the patient.

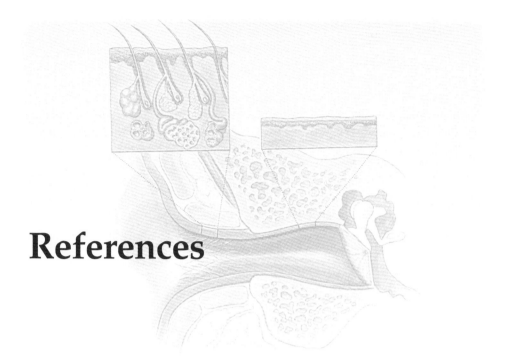

References

Adachi, B. (1937). Das Ohrenschmalz als Rassenmermal und der Rassengeruch ("Achselgeruch") nebst dem Rassenunterschied der Schweissdrusen. *Zeitshrift Rassenk, 6*, 273.

Alberti, P. W. R. M. (1964). Epithelial migration on the tympanic membrane. *Journal of Laryngology and Otology, 78*, 808–830.

Altman, F. (1950). Normal development of the ear and its mechanics. *Archives of Otolaryngology, 52*, 725.

American Speech-Language-Hearing Association. (1989). Committee on quality assurance, AIDS/HIV: Implications for speech-language pathologists and audiologists. *Asha, 31*, 33–39.

American Speech-Language-Hearing Association. (1990). Report update AIDS/HIV: Implications for speech-language pathologists and audiologists. *Asha, 32*, 46–48.

American Speech-Language-Hearing Association. (1991). External auditory canal examination and cerumen management. *Asha, 33*, 65–66.

American Speech-Language-Hearing Association. (1992). External auditory canal examination and cerumen management. Ad Hoc Committee on Advances in Clinical Practice. American Speech-Language-Hearing Association. *Asha Supplement, 6*, 22–24.

Anson, B. J. (1980). *Embryology of the ear*. Philadelphia, PA: W. B. Saunders.

Anthony, P. F., & Anthony, W. P. (1982). Surgical treatment of external auditory canal cholesteatoma. *Laryngoscope, 92*, 70–75.

Arbogast, T. (2010a). Candidacy and fitting protocols for a 24/7 hearing device. *Hearing Review, 17*(9), 34–37.

Arbogast, T. (2010b). The economics of a 24/7 hearing aid. *Hearing Review, 17*(1), 42–46.

Arbogast, T., & Whichard, S. (2009). A new hearing aid class: The first 100% invisible extended-wear hearing aid. *Hearing Review, 16*(4), 20–27.

Attal, B. S., Chang, J. J., Mathews, M. V., & Tukey, J. W. (1978). Inversion of articulatory-to-acoustic transformation in the vocal tract by computer sorting techniques. *Journal of the Acoustic Society of America, 63,* 1535–1555.

Bailes, I. H., Baird, J. W., Bari, M. A., Belletty, D. R., Bill, C. E. S., Bond, B., . . . Williams, D. T. A. (1967). Wax softening with a new preparation. *Practitioner, 199,* 359–362.

Ballachanda, B. B. (1992). Cerumen management for audiologists. *Academy of Dispensing Audiology Feedback, 3,* 21–22.

Ballachanda, B. B. (1993). Cerumen management: Causes of impaction, steps for removal. *Hearing Instruments, 44*(9), 30–33.

Ballachanda, B. B. (1995). *The human ear canal.* San Diego, CA: Singular Publishing Group.

Ballachanda, B. B. (1997). Theoretical and applied external ear acoustics. *Journal of the American Academy of Audiology, 8*(6), 411–420.

Ballachanda, B. B., & Peers, C. J. (1992). Cerumen management: Instruments and procedures. *Asha, 34,* 43–46.

Bapat, U., Nia, J., & Bance, M. (2001). Severe audiovestibular loss following ear syringing for wax removal. *Journal of Laryngology and Otology, 115*(5), 410–411.

Bass, E. J., & Jackson, J. F. (1977). Cerumen types in Eskimos. *American Journal of Physical Anthropology, 47,* 209–210.

Baxter, P. (1983). Association between use of cotton tipped swabs and cerumen plugs. *British Medical Journal (Clinical Research Ed.), 287,* 1260.

Beck, L. A. (1991). Amplification needs: Where do we go from here? In G. Studebacker, G. Bess., & L. Beck (Eds.), *The Vanderbilt hearing-aid report III* (pp. 1–9). Parkton, MD: York Press.

Bellini, M. J., Terry, R. M., & Lewis, F. A. (1989). An evaluation of common cerumenolytic agents: An in-vitro study. *Clinical Otolaryngology, 14,* 23–25.

Bende, M. (1981). Human ceruminous gland innervation. *Journal of Laryngology and Otology, 95,* 11–15.

Bentler, R. A. (1989). External ear resonance characteristics in children. *Journal of Speech and Hearing Disorders, 54,* 264–268.

Bentler, R. A. (1991). The resonance frequency of the external auditory canal in children [Letter; comment]. *Ear and Hearing, 12,* 89–90.

Bentler, R. A., & Pavlovic, C. V. (1989). Transfer functions and correction factors used in hearing aid evaluation and research. *Ear and Hearing, 10*(1), 58–63.

Berenek, L. L. (1949). *Acoustic measurements.* New York, NY: John Wily & Sons.

Berzon, D. B. (1983). Ear disease in a group general practice. A review of world communities. *Journal of Laryngology and Otology, 97,* 817–824.

Best, V., Kalluri, S., McLachlan, S., Valentine, S., Edwards, B., & Carlisle, S. (2010). A comparison of CIC and BTE hearing aids for three-dimensional localization of speech. *International Journal of Audiology, 49,* 723–732.

Bird, S. (2003). The potential pitfalls of ear syringing. Minimising the risks. *Austrian Family Physician, 32*(3), 150–151.

Bolger, J. V., Strzalkowski, C. W., & Staab, W. J. (1975). Auriculostomy, a surgical approach to hearing aid use. *Hearing Instruments, 26*(2), 14–15.

Bortz, J. T., Wertz, P. W., & Downing, D. T. (1990). Composition of cerumen lipids. *Journal of American Academy of Dermatology, 23,* 845–849.

Bradley, M. E. (1986). A new ear syringing model. *Journal of Laryngology and Otology, 100.*

Bricco, E. (1985). Impacted cerumen as a reason for failure in hearing conservation programs. *Journal of School Health, 55,* 240–241.

Brister, F., Fullwood, H. L., Ripp, T., & Blodgett, C. (1986). Incidence of occlusion due to impacted cerumen among mentally retarded adolescents. *American Journal of Mental Deficiency, 91,* 302–304.

Bruel, P., Fredricksen, E., Mathiesen, H., Rasmussen, G. Sigh, E., & Tarnow, V. (1975). Impedance of real and artificial ears. *Bruel and Kjaer Report.*

Bryant, M. P., Mueller, H. G., & Northern, J. L. (1981). Minimal contact long canal ITE hearing instruments. *Hearing Instruments, 42*(1), 12–15, 48.

Burgess, E. H. (1977). Ear wax and the right way to use an ear syringe. *Nursing Times, 73,* 1564–1565.

Burgess, E. H. (1966). A wetting agent to facilitate ear syringing. *Practitioner, 197,* 811–812.

Burkhard, M. D., & Sachs, R. M. (1975). Anthropometric manikin for acoustic research. *Journal of the Acoustical Society of America, 58,* 214–222.

Burton, M. J., & Dorée, C. J. (2009). Ear drops for the removal of earwax (Review). Cochrane Database System Review.

Caiazzo, A. J., & Tonndorf, J. (1977). Ear canal resonance and TTS. *Journal of the Acoustical Society of America, 61,* S78.

Caiazzo, A. J., & Tonndorf, J. (1978). Ear canal resonance and temporary threshold shift. *Otolaryngology, 86,* ORL-820.

Carne, S. (1980). Ear syringing. *British Medical Journal, 280,* 374–376.

Carr, M. M., & Smith R. L. (2001). Ceruminolytic efficacy in adults versus children. *Journal of Otolaryngology, 30*(3), 154–156.

Chai, T. J., & Chai, T. C. (1980). Bactericidal activity of cerumen. *Antimicrobial Agents Chemotherapy, 18,* 638–641.

Chan, J. C. K., & Giesler, C. D. (1990). Estimation of eardrum acoustic pressure and of ear canal length from remote points in the canal. *Journal of the Acoustical Society of America, 87*(3), 1237–1247.

Chandler, J. R. (1964). Partial occlusion of the external auditory meatus: Its effect upon air and bone conduction hearing acuity. *Laryngoscope, 22,* 22–54.

Chasin, M. (1995). The acoustics of CIC hearing aids. In M. Chasin (Ed.), *CIC handbook* (pp. 69–82). San Diego, CA: Singular.

Chasin, M. (In press). The acoustics of deep canal fittings. *Hearing Aid Journal.*

Cipriani, C., Taborelli, G., Gaddia, G., Melagrana, A., & Rebora, A. (1990). Production rate and composition of cerumen: Influence of sex and season. *Laryngoscope, 100,* 275–276.

Coats, A. (1974). On electrocochleographic electrode design. *Journal of the Acoustical Society of America, 56,* 708–711.

Crabtree, J. A., Britton, B. H., & Pierce, M. K. (1976). Carcinoma of the external auditory canal. *Laryngoscope, 86,* 405–415.

Craigmyle, M. B. L. (1984). *The apocrine glands and the breast*. New York, NY: John Wiley and Sons.

Crandell, C. C., & Roeser, R. J. (1993). Incidence of excessive/impacted cerumen in individuals with mental retardation: A longitudinal investigation. *American Journal of Mental Retardation, 97*, 568–574.

Cullen, J., Ellis, M., Berlin, C. I., & Lousteau, R. (1972). Human acoustic nerve action potential recording from the tympanic membrane without anesthesia. *Acta Otolaryngologica, 74*, 113–131.

Daanen, H. A. (2006). Infrared tympanic temperature and ear canal morphology. *Journal of Medical Engineering and Technology, 30*(4), 224–234.

Dahle, A. J., & McCollister, F. P. (1986). Hearing and otologic disorders in children with Down syndrome. *American Journal of Mental Deficiency, 90*, 636–642.

Delany, M. E. (1964). The acoustical impedance of human ears. *Journal of Sound and Vibration, 1*, 455–467.

Dempster, J. H., & Mackenzie, K. (1990). The resonance frequency of the external auditory canal in children [See comments]. *Ear and Hearing, 11*, 296–298.

DeWeese, D., & Saunders, W. (1973). *Otolaryngology* (4th ed.). St. Louis, MO: Mosby.

DiBartolomeo, J. R. (1979). Exostoses of the external auditory canal. *Annals of Otology Rhinology and Laryngology Supplement, 88*, 2–20.

Dillon, H., James, A., & Ginis, J. (1997). Client Oriented Scale of Improvement (COSI) and its relationship to several other measures of benefit and satisfaction provided by hearing aids. *Journal of the American Academy of Audiology, 8*(1), 27–43.

Dinsdale, R. C., Roland, P. S., Manning, S. C., & Meyerhoff, W. L. (1991). Catastrophic otologic injury from oral jet irrigation of the external auditory canal. *Laryngoscope, 101*, 75–78.

Dirks, D. D., & Kincaid, G. E. (1987). Basic acoustic considerations of ear canal probe measurements. *Ear and Hearing, 8*, 60S–67S.

Djupesland, G., & Zwislocki, J. J. (1972). Sound pressure distribution in the outer ear. *Scandinavian Audiology, 4*, 197–203.

Driscoll, P. V., Ramachandrula, A., Drezner, D. A., Hicks, T. A., & Schaffer, S. R. (1993). Characteristics of cerumen in diabetic patients: A key to understanding malignant external otitis. *Otolaryngology-Head and Neck Surgery, 109*, 676–679.

Eckerdal, O., Ahlqvist, J., Alehagen, U., & Wing, K. (1978). Length dimensions and morphologic variations of the external bony auditory canal. *Dentomaxillofacial Radiology, 7*, 43–50.

Edwards, J., & Harris, K. S. (1990). Rotation and translation of the jaw during speech. *Journal of Speech and Hearing Research, 33*, 550–562.

Egolf, D. P., Nelson, D. K., Howell, H. C. I., & Larson, V. D. (1993). Quantifying ear-canal geometry with multiple computer-assisted tomographic scans. *Journal of the Acoustical Society of America, 93*(5), 2809–2819.

Ernst, E. (2004). Ear candles: A triumph of ignorance over science. *Journal of Laryngology and Otology, 118*, 1–2.

Fahmey, S., & Whitefield, M. (1982). Multicentre clinical trial of Exerol as a cerumenolytic. *British Journal of Clinical Practice, 36,* 197–204.

Farmer-Fedor, B. L., Rabbitt, R. D. (2002). Acoustic intensity, impedance and reflection coefficient in the human ear canal. *Journal of the Acoustical Society of America, 112,* 600–620.

Ford, G. R., & Courteney-Harris, R. G. (1990). Another hazard of ear syringing: Malignant external otitis. *Journal of Laryngology and Otology, 104,* 709–710.

Fortune, T. W., & Preves, D. A. (1992). Hearing aid saturation and aided loudness discomfort. *Journal of Speech and Hearing Research, 35,* 175–185.

Fraden, J. (1991). The development of Thermoscan Instant Thermometer. *Clinical Pediatrics (Philadelphia), 30,* 11–2; discussion 34–35.

Fraser, J. G. (1970). The efficacy of wax solvents: In vitro studies and a clinical trial. *Journal of Laryngology and Otology, 84,* 1055–1064.

Freedman, A. (1990). The efficacy of ceruminolytics [Letter; comment]. *Journal of Otolaryngology, 19,* 150–151.

Freeman, R. B.(1995). Impacted cerumen: How to safely remove earwax in an office visit. *Geriatrics, 50,* 52–53.

Gerhardt, K. J., Rodriguez, G. P., Helper, E. L., & Moul, M. L. (1987). Ear canal volume and variability in the pattern of temporary threshold shifts. *Ear and Hearing, 8,* 316–321.

Gibbons, L. V. (1967). Body temperature monitoring in the external auditory meatus. *Aerospace Medicine, 38*(7), 671–675.

Gilman, S., & Dirks, D. D. (1986). Acoustics of ear canal measurement of eardrum SPL in simulators. *Journal of the Acoustical Society of America, 80,* 783–793.

Ginsberg, I. A., & White, T. P. (1985). Otological consideration in audiology. In J. Katz (Ed.), *Handbook of clinical audiology* (3rd ed.). Baltimore, MD: William & Wilkins.

Gleitman, R. M., Ballachanda, B. B., & Goldstein, D. P. (1992). Incidence of cerumen impaction in general adult population. *Hearing Journal, 45,* 28–32.

Graber, R. F. (1986). Removing impacted cerumen. *Patient Care, 20,* 151–153.

Grossan, M. (1978). A new ear irrigator. *Archives of Otorhino-laryngology, 86,* 936–937.

Grossan, M. (1998). Cerumen removal—current challenges. *Ear Nose and Throat Journal, 77*(7), 541–546.

Gudmundsen, G. I. (1994). Fitting CIC hearing aids—some practical pointers. *Hearing Journal, 47*(7), 44–47.

Guest, J. F., Greener, M. J., Robinson, A. C., & Smith, A. F. (2004). Impacted cerumen: Composition, production, epidemiology and management. *QJM, 97*(8), 477–488.

Gulya, A. J. (1990). Developmental anatomy of the ear. In M. E. Glasscock, III, G. E. Shambuagh, & G. D. Johnson (Eds.), *Surgery of the ear* (pp. 5–33). Philadelphia, PA: W. B. Saunders.

Hand, C., & Harvey, I. (2004). The effectiveness of topical preparations for the treatment of earwax: A systematic review. *British Journal of General Practice, 54,* 862–867.

Harvey, D. J (1989). Identification of long-chain fatty acids and alcohols from human cerumen by the use of picolinyl and nicotinate esters. *Biomedical Environmental Mass Spectrometry, 18,* 719–723.

Hawke, M., Knie, M., & Alberti, P. W. (1990). *Clinical otoscopy: A text and color atlas.* New York, NY: Churchill Livingstone.

Hellstrom, P. A., & Axelsson, A. (1993). Miniature microphone probe tube measurements in the external auditory canal. *Journal of the Acoustical Society of America, 93,* 907–919.

Hinchcliffe, R. (1955). Efficacy of current cerumenolytics. *British Medical Journal, 17*(2), 722.

His, W. (1885). Torisieme cong. internat. d'otologie. *Compte Rend Bale, 149.*

Hollinshead, W. H. (1968*). Anatomy for surgeons: Vol. 1: The head and neck.* New York, NY: Harper and Row.

Holt, J. J. (1992). Ear canal cholesteatoma. *Laryngoscope, 102,* 608–613.

Hudde, H. (1983). Estimation of the area function of human ear canal by sound pressure measurements. *Journal of the Acoustical Society of America, 73,* 24–31.

Hudde, H., & Schmidt, S. (2009). Sound fields in generally shaped curved ear canals. *Journal of the Acoustical Society of America, 125*(5), 3146–3157.

Hyslop, N. E. (1971). Earwax and host defense. *New England Journal of Medicine, 284,* 1099–1100.

Ibraimov, A. I. (1991). Cerumen phenotypes in certain populations of Eurasia and Africa. *American Journal of Physical Anthropology, 84,* 209–211.

Inaba, M., Chung, T. H., Kim, J. C., Choi, Y. C., & Kim, J. H. (1987). Lipid composition of ear wax in hircismus. *Yonsei Medical Journal, 28,* 49–51.

Johansen, P. A. (1975). Measurement of the human ear canal. *Acoustica, 33,* 349–351.

Johnson, A., & Hawke, M. (1988). The non auditory physiology of the external ear. In A. F. Jahn & J. Santo-Sachi (Eds.), *Physiology of the ear.* New York, NY: Raven Press.

Johnson, S. E., & Nelson, P. B. (1991). Real ear measures of auditory brainstem response click spectra in infants and adults. *Ear and Hearing, 12,* 180–183.

Kalcioglu, M. T., Durmaz, R., Ozturan, O., Bayindir, Y., & Direkel, S. (2004). Does cerumen have a risk for transmission of hepatitis B? *Laryngoscope, 114*(3), 577–580.

Keane, E. M., Wilson, H., McGrane, D., Coakley, D., & Walsh, J. B. (1995). Use of solvents to disperse ear wax. *British Journal of Clinical Practice, 49*(2), 71–72.

Keefe, D. H., Bulen, J. C., Campbell, S. L., & Burns, E. M. (1994). Pressure transfer function and absorption cross-section from the diffuse field to the human infant ear canal. *Journal of the Acoustical Society of America, 95,* 355–371.

Keller, A. P. J. (1958). Study of the relationship of air pressure to myringorupture. *Laryngoscope, 68,* 2015–2029.

Kemink, J. L., & Graham, M. D. (1982). Osteomas and exostoses of the external auditory canal—medical and surgical management. *Journal of Otolaryngology, 11*(2), 101–106.

Kenna, M .A. (1990). Embryology and developmental anatomy of the ear. In C. Bluestone, S. Stool, & M. Scheetz (Eds.), *Pediatric Otolaryngology* (2nd ed, pp. 77–80). Philadelphia, PA: W. B. Saunders.

Khanna, S. M., & Stinson, M. R. (1985). Specification of the acoustical input to the ear at high frequencies. *Journal of the Acoustical Society of America, 77,* 577–589.

Killion, M. C., Wilber, L. A., & Gudmundsen, G. (1988). Zwislocki was right . . . a potential solution to the "hollow voice" problem (the amplified occlusion effect) with deeply sealed earmolds. *Hearing Instruments, 39,* 1, 14.

Kochkin, S. (2010) MarkeTrak VIII: Consumer satisfaction with hearing aids is slowly increasing. *Hearing Journal, 63*(1), 19–32.

Kruger, B. (1987). An update on the external ear resonance in infants and young children. *Ear and Hearing, 8,* 333–336.

Kurosumi, K., & Kawabata, I. (1976). Transmission and scanning electron microscopy of the human ceruminous apocrine gland. I .Secretory glandular cells. *Archives of Histology Japan, 39,* 207–229.

Larsen, G. (1976). Removing cerumen with a water pik. *American Journal of Nursing, 76*(2), 264–265.

Lawton, B. W., & Stinson, M. R. (1986). Standing wave patterns in the human ear canal used for estimation of acoustic energy reflectance at the eardrum. *Journal of the Acoustical Society of America, 79,* 1003–1009.

Lewis-Cullinan, C., & Janken, J. K. (1990). Effect of cerumen removal on the hearing ability of geriatric patients. *Journal of Advanced Nursing, 15,* 594–600.

Lum, C.L., Jeyanthi, S., Prepagerna, N., Vadivelu, J., Raman, R. (2009). Antibacterial and antifungal properties of human cerumen. *The Journal of Laryngology & Otology, 123,*375–378.

Lybarger, S. F. (1978). Expanding the usefulness of adjustable vent inserts. *Hearing Instruments, 29,* 18–19.

Lynde, C. W., McLean, D. I., & Wood, W. S. (1984). Tumors of ceruminous glands. *Journal of American Academy of Dermatology, 11,* 841–847.

Lyndon, S., Roy, P., Grillage, M. G., & Miller, A. J. (1992). A comparison of the efficacy of two ear drop preparations ("Audax" and "Earex") in the softening and removal of impacted ear wax. *Current Medical Research and Opinion, 13*(1), 21–25.

Macknin, M. L., Talo, H., & Medendrop, S. V. (1994). Effect of cotton-tipped swab use on ear-wax occlusion. *Clinical Pediatrics (Philadelphia), 33,* 14–18.

Macrae, J., & Dillon, H. (1996). Gain, frequency response and maximum output requirements for hearing aids. *Journal of Rehabilitation Research and Development, 33*(4), 363–376.

Mahoney, D. F. (1987). One simple solution to hearing impairment. *Geriatric Nursing (New York), 8*(85), 242–245.

Mahoney, D. F. (1993). Cerumen impaction. Prevalence and detection in nursing homes. *Journal of Gerontological Nursing, 19,* 23–30.

Main, T., & Lim, D. (1976). The human external auditory canal—an ultrastructural study. *Laryngoscope, 86,* 1164–1176.

Mandour, M. A., El-Ghazzawi, E. F., Toppozada, H. H., & Malaty, H. A. (1974). Histological and histochemical study of the activity of ceruminous glands in normal and excessive wax accumulation. *Journal of Laryngology and Otology, 11,* 1175–1085.

Marshall, K. G., & Attia, E. L. (1983). *Disorders of the ear.* Boston, MA: John Wright — PSG.

Matsunaga, E. (1962). The dimorphism in human normal cerumen. *Annals of Human Genetics, London, 25,* 273–286.

Mawson, S. R. (1974). Middle ear effusions: Therapy and clinical results. *Annals of Otology, Rhinology, and Laryngology, 83*(Suppl. 11), 71–72.

McCarter, D. F., Courtney, A. U., & Pollart, S. M. (2007). Cerumen impaction. *American Family Physician, 75*(10), 1523–1528.

McMillan, M. D., & Willette, J. (1988). Aseptic technique: A procedure for preventing disease transmission in the practice environment. *Asha, 30,* 35–37.

Meehan, P., Isenhour, J. L., Reeves, R., et al. (2002). Ceruminolysis in the pediatric patient: A prospective, double-blinded, randomized controlled trial. *Academic Emergency Medicine, 9,* 521–522.

Megarry, S., Pett, A., Scarlett, A., Teh, W., Zeigler, E., & Canter, R. J. (1988). The activity against yeasts of human cerumen. *Journal of Laryngology and Otology, 102,* 671–672.

Mehrgardt, S., & Mellert, V. (1977). Transformation characteristics of the external human ear. *Journal of the Acoustical Society of America, 61,* 1567–1576.

Meikle, M. B., Stewart, B. J., Griest, S. E., Martin, W. H., Henry, J. A., Abrams, H. B., . . . Sandridge, S. A. (2007). Assessment of tinnitus: Measurement of treatment outcomes. *Progress in Brain Research, 166,* 511–521.

Middlebrooks, J. C. (1992). Narrow-band sound localization related to external ear acoustics. *Journal of the Acoustical Society of America, 92,* 2607–2624.

Middlebrooks, J. C. (1999a). Individual differences in external-ear transfer functions reduced by scaling in frequency. *Journal of the Acoustical Society of America, 106,* 1480–1492.

Middlebrooks, J. C. (1999b). Virtual localization improved by scaling nonindividualized external-ear transfer functions in frequency. *Journal of the Acoustical Society of America Society of America, 106,* 1493–1510.

Middlebrooks, J. C., Makous, J. C., & Green, D. M. (1989). Directional sensitivity of sound-pressure levels in the human ear canal. *Journal of the Acoustical Society of America, 86,* 89–107.

Miura, K., Yoshiura, K., Miura, S., Shimada, T., Yamasaki, K., Yoshida, A., . . . Masuzaki, H. (2007). A strong association between human earwax-type and apocrine colostrum secretion from the mammary gland. *Human Genetics, 121*(5), 631–633.

Montagna, W., & Parakkal, P. F. (1974). *The structure and function of skin* (3rd ed.). New York, NY: Academic Press.

Morton, J. Y., & Jones, R. A. (1956). The acoustical impedance presented by some human ears to hearing aid earphones of insert type. *Acoustica, 6,* 339–345.

Moryl, C., Danhauer, J., & Di Bartolomeo. (1992). Real ear unaided responses in ears with tympanic membrane perforations. *Journal of the American Academy of Audiology, 3*, 60–65.

Musicant, A. D., Chan, J. C. K., & Hind, J. E. (1990). Direction-dependent spectral properties of cat external ear: New data and cross-species comparisons. *Journal of the Acoustical Society of America, 87*, 757–781.

Mueller, H. G., & Hall, J. (1998). *Audiology desk reference, Volume II*. San Diego, CA: Singular.

Muller, G. H., Hawkins, D. B., & Northern, J. L. (1992). *Probe microphone measurements*. San Diego, CA: Singular.

Myers, B. A., Siegfried, M., & Pueschel, S. M. (1987). Pseudodementia in the mentally retarded. A case report and review. *Clinical Pediatrics (Philadelphia), 26*, 275–277.

Naeve, S. L., Margolis, R. H., Levine, S. C., & Fournier, E. M. (1992). Effect of ear canal air pressure on evoked otoacoustic emissions. *Journal of the Acoustical Society of America, 4*, 2091–2095.

Nishimura, Y., & Kumoi, T. (1992). The embryologic development of the human external auditory meatus. Preliminary report. *Acta Otolaryngologica (Stockholm), 112*, 496–503.

Northern, J. L., & Downs, M. P. (1992). *Hearing in children* (4th ed.). Baltimore, MD: Williams & Wilkins.

Ohashi, J., Naka, I., & Tsuchiya, N. (2011). The impact of natural selection on an ABCC11 SNP determining earwax type. *Molecular Biology and Evolution, 28*, 849–857.

Okuda, I., Bingham, B., Stoney, P., & Hawke, M. (1991). The organic composition of earwax. *Journal of Otolaryngology, 20*, 212–215.

Osborne, J. E., & Baty, J. D. (1990). Do patients with otitis externa produce biochemically different cerumen? *Clinical Otolaryngology, 15*, 59–61.

Pearlman, R. C., & Hoffman, S. R. (1976). Basic considerations of otoscopic technique. *Maico Audiological Library Series, 15*(7), 1–3.

Perry, E. T. (1957). *The human ear canal*. Springfield, IL: Charles C. Thomas.

Perry, E. T., & Nichols, A. C. (1956). Studies on the growth of bacteria in the human ear canal. *Journal of Investigative Dermatology, 27*, 165–170.

Petrakis, N. L. (1969). Dry cerumen—a prevalent genetic trait among American Indians. *Nature, 222*, 1080–1081.

Petrakis, N. L. (1971). Cerumen genetics and human breast cancer. *Science, 173*, 347–349.

Petrakis, N. L. (1983). Cerumen phenotype and epithelial dysplasia in nipple aspirates of breast fluid. *American Journal of Physical Anthropology, 62*, 115–118.

Petrakis, N. L., Ernster, V. L., Sacks, S. T., King, E. B., Schweitzer, R. J., Hunt, T. K., & King, M. C. (1981). Epidemiology of breast fluid secretion: Association with breast cancer risk factors and cerumen type. *Journal of National Cancer Institute, 67*, 277–284.

Petrakis, N. L., King, E. B., Lee, M., & Miike, R. (1990). Cerumen phenotype and proliferative epithelium in breast fluids of U.S.-born vs. immigrant Asian women: A possible genetic-environmental interaction. *Breast Cancer Research Treatment, 16,* 279–285.

Petrakis, N. L., Lowenstein, J. M., Wiencke, J. K., Lee, M. M., Wrensch, M. R., King, E. B., . . . Miike, R. (1993). Gross cystic disease fluid protein in nipple aspirates of breast fluid of Asian and non-Asian women. *Cancer Epidemiology Biomarkers Prevention, 2,* 573–579.

Petrakis, N. L., Mason, L., Lee, R. E., Sugimoto, B., Pawson, S., & Catchpool, F. (1975). Association of race, age, menopausal status, and cerumen type with breast fluid secretion in nonlactating women as determined by nipple aspiration. *Journal of National Cancer Institute, 54,* 829–834.

Petrakis, N. L., Molohon, K. T., & Tepper, D. J. (1967). Cerumen in American Indians: Genetic implications of sticky and dry types. *Science, 158,* 1192–1193.

Petrakis, N. L., Pringle, U., Petrakis, S. J., & Petrakis, S. L. (1971). Evidence for a genetic cline in ear wax types in the Middle East and Southeast Asia. *American Journal of Physical Anthropology, 35,* 141–144.

Pierson, L. L., Gerhardt, K. J., Rodriguez, G. P., & Yanke, R. B. (1994). Relationship between outer ear resonance and permanent noise-induced hearing loss. *American Journal of Otolaryngology, 15,* 37–40.

Prasad, K. S. (1984). Cardiac depression on syringing the ear: A case report. *Journal of Laryngology and Otology, 98,* 1013.

Preves, D. (1994). Real-ear gain provided by CIC, ITC and ITE hearing instruments. *Hearing Review, 1*(7), 61–80.

Preves, D. A., & Woodruff, B .D. (1990). Some methods of improving and assessing hearing aid headroom. *Audecibel, 38,* 8–13.

Qi, L., Liu, H., Lutfy, J., Funnell, W. R., &, S. J. (2006). A nonlinear finite-element model of the newborn ear canal. *Journal of the Acoustical Society of America, 120,* 3789–3798.

Rabbitt, R. D. (1990). A hierarchy of examples illustrating the acoustic coupling of the eardrum. *Journal of the Acoustical Society of America, 87,* 2566–2582.

Rabbitt, R. D., & Friedrich, M. T. (1991). Ear canal cross-sectional pressure distributions: Mathematical analysis and computation. *Journal of the Acoustical Society of America, 89*(5), 2379–2390.

Rabbitt, R. D., & Holmes, M. H. (1989). Three-dimensional acoustic waves in the ear canal and their interaction with the tympanic membrane. *Journal of the Acoustical Society of America, 83,* 1064–1080.

Rabinowitz, W. (1977). *On the input acoustic admittance of the human middle ear.* (Unpublished doctoral dissertation). Massachusettes Institute of Technology, Cambridge, MA.

Rafferty, J., Tsikoudas, A., & Davis, B. C. (2007). Ear candling: Should general practitioners recommend it? *Canadian Family Physician, 53*(12), 2121–2122.

Raman, R. (1986). Impacted ear wax—a cause for unexplained cough? [Letter]. *Archivea of Otolaryngology-Head and Neck Surgery, 112,* 679.

Rasetshwane, D. M., & Neely, S. T. (2011). Inverse solution of ear-canal area function from reflectance. *Journal of the Acoustical Society of America, 130*(6), 3873–3881.

Ress, B. D., Luntz, M., Telischi, F. F., Balkany, T. J., & Whiteman, M. L. (1997). Necrotizing external otitis in patients with AIDS. *Laryngoscope, 107*, 456–460.

Ricketts, T., Johnson, E., & Federmna, J. (2008.) Individual differences within and across feedback suppression hearing aids. *Journal of the American Academy of Audiology, 19,* 748–757.

Robinson, A. C., & Hawke, M. (1989). The efficacy of ceruminolytics: Everything old is new again [see comments]. *Journal of Otolaryngology, 18,* 263–267.

Robinson, A. C., Hawke, M., MacKay, A., Ekem, J. K., & Stratis, M. (1989). The mechanism of ceruminolysis. *Journal of Otolaryngology, 18,* 268–273.

Robinson, A. C., Hawke, M., & Naiberg, J. (1990). Impacted cerumen: A disorder of keratinocyte separation in the superficial external ear canal? *Journal of Otolaryngology, 19,* 86–90.

Roche, A. F., Siervogel, R .M., & Himes, J. H. (1978). Longitudinal study of hearing in children: Baseline data concerning auditory thresholds, noise exposure and biological factors. *Journal of the Acoustical Society of America, 64,* 1593–1601.

Rodriguez, G. P., & Gerhardt, K. J. (1991). Influence of outer ear resonant frequency on patterns of temporary threshold shift. *Ear and Hearing, 12,* 110–114.

Roeser, R. J., Adams, R. M., Roland, P., & Wilson, P. L. (1992). A safe and effective procedure for cerumen management. *Audiology Today, 4,* 26–30.

Roeser, R. J., Adams, R. M., & Watkins, S. (1991). Cerumen management in hearing conservation: The Dallas (Texas) Independent School District program. *Journal of School Health, 61,* 47–49.

Roeser, R. J., & Ballachanda, B. B. (1997). Physiology, pathophysiology, and anthropology/epidemiology of human earcanal secretions. *Journal of the American Academy of Audiology, 8*(6), 391–400.

Roeser, R. J., & Crandell, C. (1991). More on "The Responsibility of Audiologists in Cerumen Management." *Audiology Today, 3*(3), 20–21.

Roeser, R. J., & Roland, P. (1992). What audiologists must know about cerumen and cerumen management. *American Journal of Audiology,* 27–34.

Roland, P. S., Smith, T. L., Schwartz, S. R., Rosenfeld, R. M., Ballachanda, B., Earll, J. M., . . . Wetmore, S. (2008). Clinical practice guideline: Cerumen impaction. *Otolaryngology-Head and Neck Surgery, 139*(3 Suppl. 2), S1–S21.

Rubel, E .W., Born, D. E., Dietch, J. S., & Durham, D. (1984). Recent advances toward understanding auditory system development. In C. I. Berlin (Ed.), *Hearing science* (pp. 109–158). San Diego, CA: College-Hill Press.

Rubin, J., & Yu, V. L. (1988). Malignant external otitis: Insights into pathogenesis, clinical manifestations, diagnosis, and therapy. *American Journal of Medicine, 85,* 391–398.

Rubin, J., Yu, V. L., Kamerer, D. B., & Wagener, M. (1990). Aural irrigation with water: A potential pathogenic mechanism for inducing malignant external otitis? *Annals of Otology, Rhinology, and Laryngology, 99,* 117–119.

Ruby, R. R. (1986). Conductive hearing loss in the elderly. *Journal of Otolaryngology, 15,* 245–247.

Salomon, J. L. (1967). New technique for rapid ear irrigations. *Journal of Occupational Medicine, 9,* 576–577.

Salvinelli, F., Maurizi, M., Calamita, S., D'Alatri, L., Capelli, A., & Carbone, A. (1991). The external ear and the tympanic membrane: A three-dimensional study. *Scandinavian Audiology, 20,* 253–256.

Sandridge, S. A., & Newman, C. W. (2006, March 6). Improving the efficiency and accountability of the hearing aid selection process—use of the COAT. *AudiologyOnline* (accessed December 14, 2012).

Scherl, M., Szabo, D., Desai, N., Scherl, S., Whichard, S., & Arbogast, T. (2011). Real-world safety experience with a 24/7 hearing device. *Hearing Review, 18*(1), 18–23.

Schwartz, R. H., Rodriguez, W. J., McAveney, W., & Grundfast, K. M. (1983). Cerumen removal. How necessary is it to diagnose acute otitis media? *American Journal of Diseases of Children, 137,* 1064–1065.

Seewald, R., Cornelisse, L., Richert, F., & Block, M. (1995). Acoustic transforms for fitting CIC instruments. In M. Chasin (Ed.), *The CIC handbook.* San Diego, CA: Singular.

Senturia, B. H. (1976). *Diffuse external otitis: Current guide to pathogenesis, diagnosis, management.* A Wellcome Medical Education Service.

Shanks, J. E., & Lilly, D. J. (1981). An evaluation of tympanometric estimates of ear canal volume. *Journal of Speech and Hearing Research, 24,* 557–566.

Sharp, J. F., Wilson, J. A., Ross, L., & Barr Hamilton, R. M. (1990). Ear wax removal: A survey of current practice. *British Medical Journal, 301,* 1251–1253.

Shaw, E. A. G. (1966). Earcanal pressure generated by a free sound field. *Journal of the Acoustical Society of America, 39,* 465–470.

Shaw, E. A. G. (1969). Hearing threshold and ear-canal pressure levels with varying acoustic field. *Journal of the Acoustical Society of America, 46,* 1502–1514.

Shaw, E. A. G. (1974a). The external ear. In W. D. Keidel & W. D. Neff (Eds.), *Handbook of sensory physiology, Vol. 1, Auditory system* (pp. 455–490). New York, NY: Springer Verlag.

Shaw, E. A. G. (1974b). Transformation of sound pressure level from the free field to the eardrum in the horizontal plane. *Journal of the Acoustical Society of America, 56,* 1848–1860.

Shaw, E. A. G. (1975). The external ear: New knowledge. In S. C. Dalsgaard (Ed), Earmold and associated problems. *Proceedings of the Seventh Danavox Symposium. Scandinavian Audiology Suppl., 5,* 24–50.

Shaw, E. A. G. (1980). The acoustics of the external ear. In G. A. Studebaker & I. Hochberg (Eds.), *Acoustical factors affecting hearing aid performance and measurement.* Baltimore, MD: University Park Press.

Shaw, E. A .G., & Teranishi, R. (1968). Sound pressure generated in an external-ear replica and real human ears by a nearby point source. *Journal of the Acoustical Society of America, 44*(1), 240–249.

Shaw, E. A. G., & Villancourt, M. M. (1985). Transformation of sound-pressure level from the free field to the eardrum presented in numerical form. *Journal of Acoustical Society of America, 78,* 1120–1123.

Sheehy, J. L. (1982). Diffuse exostoses and osteomata of the external auditory canal: A report of 100 operations. *Otolaryngology-Head and Neck Surgery, 90,* 337–342.

Shichijo, S., Masuda, H., & Takeuchi, M. (1979). Carbohydrate composition of glycopetides from the human cerumen. *Biochemical Medicine, 22,* 256–263.

Shugyo, Y., Sudo, N., Kanai, K., Yamashita, T., Kumazawa, T., & Kanamura, S. (1988). Morphological differences between secretory cells of wet and dry types of human ceruminous glands. *American Journal of Anatomy, 181,* 377–384.

Siegel, J. H. (1994). Ear-canal standing waves and high frequency sound calibration using otoacoustic emission probes. *Journal of the Acoustical Society of America, 95,* 2589–2597.

Sim, D. W. (1988). Wax plugs and cotton buds. *Journal of Laryngology and Otology, 102,* 575–576.

Simonetta, B., & Magnoni, A. (1937). Lo siviluppo delle ghialndole sebacee ceruminose del condotto uditivo esterno nell'umo. *Archivio Italiano di Anatomia e di Embriologia, 39,* 245–261.

Singer, D. E., Freeman, E., Hoffert, W. R., Keys, R. J., Mitchell, R. B., & Hardy, A. V. (1952). Otitis externa: bacteriological and mycological studies. *Annals of Otology, Rhinology and Laryngology, 61,* 317–330.

Singer, A. J., Sauris, E., & Viccellio, A. W. (2000). Ceruminolytic effects of docusate sodium: A randomized, controlled trial. *Annals of Emergency Medicine, 36*(3), 228–232.

Smelt, G., Hawke, M., & Proops, D. (1988). Anatomy of the external ear canal: A new technique for making impressions. *Journal of Otolaryngology, 17,* 249–253.

Somerville, G. (2002). The most effective products available to facilitate ear syringing. *British Journal of Community Nursing, 7,* 94–101.

Sondhi, M. M., & Gopinath, B. (1971). Determination of vocal-tract shape from impulse response at the lips. *Journal of the Acoustical Society of America, 49,* 1867–1873.

Sooy, C. D., Gerberding, J. L., & Kaplan, M. J. (1987). The risk for otolaryngologists who treat patients with aids and aids virus infection: Report of an in-process study. *Laryngoscope, 97,* 430–434.

Sperber, G. H. (1994). Embryology of the head and neck. In G. M. English (Ed.), *Otolarngology, plastic and reconstructive surgery* (4th ed.). Philadelphia, PA: J. B. Lippincott.

Staab, W. J. (1989 September). *Deep canal hearing aids: A fitting rationale.* American Auditory Society 16th Annual Meeting, New Orleans, LA.

Staab, W. J. (1993). Precipitous, high-frequency hearing losses: A new solution. *Hearing Instruments, 44*(4), 20–22.

Staab, W. J. (1995). Deep canal hearing aids. In B. Ballachanda (Ed.), *The human ear canal* (pp. 27–52). San Diego, CA: Singular Publishing Group.

Staab, W. J. (1997). Introduction to deep canal principles. *Seminars in Hearing, 17*(1), 3–20.

Staab, W. J., & Finlay, B. (1991). A fitting rationale for deep canal hearing instruments. *Hearing Instruments, 42*(1), 6–10, 48.

Stinson, M. R. (1985). The spatial distribution of sound pressure within scaled replicas of the human ear canal. *Journal of the Acoustical Society of America, 78,* 1596–1602.

Stinson, M. R., & Daigle, G. A. (2005). Comparison of an analytic horn equation approach and a boundary element method for the calculation of sound fields in the human ear canal. *Journal of the Acoustical Society of America, 118,* 2405–2411.

Stinson, M. R., & Daigle, G. A. (2007). Transverse pressure distributions in a simple model ear canal occluded by a hearing aid test fixture. *Journal of the Acoustical Society of America, 121*(6), 3689–3702.

Stinson, M. R., & Khann, S. M. (1994). Spatial distribution of sound pressure and energy flow in the ear canals of cats. *Journal of the Acoustical Society of America, 96,* 170–180.

Stinson, M .R., & Lawton, B. W. (1989). Specification of the geometry of the human ear canal for the prediction of sound-pressure level distribution. *Journal of the Acoustical Society of America, 85,* 2492–2503.

Stinson, M. R., & Shaw, E. A. G. (1983). Sound pressure distribution in the human ear canal. *Journal of the Acoustical Society of America, 73,* 559–560.

Stinson, M. R., Shaw, E. A. G., & Lawton, B. W. (1982). Estimation of acoustical energy reflectance at the eardrum from measurements of pressure distribution in the human ear canal. *Journal of the Acoustical Society of America, 72,* 766–773.

Stoeckelhuber, M., Matthias, C., Andratschke, M., Stoeckelhuber, B. M., Koehler, C., Herzmann, S., . . . Welschhuman., U. (2006). Ceruminous gland: Ultrastructure and histochemical analysis of antimicrobial and cytoskeletal components. *The Anatomical Record Part A, 288A,* 877–884.

Stone, M., & Fulghum, R. S. (1984). Bactericidal activity of wet cerumen. *Annals of Otology, Rhinology, and Laryngology, 93,* 183–186.

Storrs, L. A. (1981). Management of the ear canal seborrhea with cerumen. *Laryngoscope, 91,* 1231–1233.

Streeter, G. L. (1922). Development of the auricle in the human embryo. *Contribution to Embryology, 14,* 111.

Stypulkowski, P., & Staller, S. (1987). Clinical evaluation of a new ECoG recording electrode. *Ear and Hearing, 8,* 304–310.

Teranishi, R., & Shaw, E. A. G. (1968). External-ear acostic models with simple geometry. *Journal of the Acoustical Society of America, 44,* 257–263.

Testa-Riva, F., & Puxeddu, P. (1980). Secretory mechanisms of human ceruminous glands: A transmission and scanning electron microscopic study. *Anatomical Record, 196,* 363–372.

Thibodeau, L. (2004). Maximizing communication via hearing assistance technology: Plotting beyond the audiogram. *Hearing Journal, 57*, 46–51.

Tomita, H., Yamada, K., Ghadami, M., Oqura, T., Yanai, Y., Nakatomi, K., . . . Nikawa, N. (2002). Mapping of the wet/dry earwax locus to the pericentromeric region of chromosome 16. *Lancet, 359*, 2000–2002.

Toyoda, Y., Sakurai, A., Mitani, Y. Nakashima, M., Yoshiura, K., Nakagawa, H., . . . Toshihisa, I. (2009). Earwax, osmidrosis, and breast cancer: Why does one SNP (538G>A) in the human ABC transporter *ABCC11* gene determine earwax type? *FASEB Journal, 23*(6), 2001–2013.

Twerenbold, R., Zehnder, A., Breidthardt, T., Reichlin, T., Reiter, M., Schaub, N., . . . Mueller, C. (2010). Limitations of infrared ear temperature measurement in clinical practice. *Swiss Medical Weekly, 20*, 140. w13131. doi:10.4414/smw.2010.13131

Van De Water, T. R., Maderson, P. F. A., & Jaskoll, T. F. (1980). The morphogenesis of the middle and external ear. *Birth Defects, 16*(4), 147.

Van De Water, T. R., Maderson, P. F. A., & Jaskoll, T. F. (1988). Embryology of the ear, outer, middle, and inner. In P. W. Alberti & R. J. Ruben (Eds.), *Otologic medicine and surgery* (pp. 3–27). New York, NY: Churchill Livingstone.

Van Vliet, D., & Galster, J. (2010). *Invisible-in-the-canal (IIC) hearing aids*. Starkey Whitepaper.

Van Willigen, J. (1976). Some morphological aspects of the meatus acusticus externus in connection with mandibular movements. *Journal of Oral Rehabilitation, 3*, 299–304.

Varoba, B. (1987). Patient-selected soft canal hearing instruments. *Hearing Instruments, 38*(4), 39.

Virapongse, C., Sarwar, M., Sasaki, C., & Kier, E. L. (1983). High resolution computed tomography of the osseous external auditory canal: 1. Normal anatomy. *Journal of Computer Assisted Tomography, 7*(3), 486–492.

Warwick-Brown, N. P. (1986). Wax impaction in the ear. *Practitioner, 230*, 301.

Watkins, S., Moore, T. H., & Phillips, J. (1984). Clearing impacted ears. *American Journal of Nursing, 84*(110), 1107.

Weinroth, S. E., Schessel, D., & Tuazon, C. U. (1994). Malignant otitis externa in AIDS patients: Case report and review of the literature. *Ear Nose and Throat Journal, 73*, 777–778.

Whatley, V. N., Dodds, C. L., & Paul, R. I. (2003). Randomized clinical trial of docusate, triethanolamine polypeptide, and irrigation in cerumen removal in children. *Archives of Pediatric and Adolescent Medicine, 157*(12), 1177–1180.

Wiener, F. M., & Ross, D. A. (1946). The pressure distribution in the auditory canal in a progressive sound field. *Journal of the Acoustical Society of America, 18*, 401–408.

William, G. H. (1988). Developmental anatomy of the ear. In G. M.English (Ed.), *Diseases of the ear and hearing* (Rev. ed., pp. 1–67). Philadelphia, PA: J. B. Lippincott.

William, R. J., & Thompson, R. C. (1948). A device for obtaining a continuous record of body temperature from the external auditory canal. *Science, 90*, 190.

Wilson, S. A., & Lopez, R. (2002). Clinical inquiries. What is the best treatment for impacted cerumen. *Journal of Family Practice, 51,* 117.

Wood-Jones, F., & Wen, I. (1934). The development of the external ear. *Journal of Anatomy, 68,* 525–533.

Woodburne, R. T. (1978). *Essentials of human anatomy* (6th ed.). New York, NY: Oxford University Press.

Wright, C. G. (1997). Development of the human external ear. *Journal of the American Academy of Audiology, 8*(6), 379–390.

Yaron, M., Lowenstein, S. R., & Koziol-McLain, J. (1995). Measuring the accuracy of the infrared tympanic thermometer: Correlation does not signify agreement. *Journal of Emergency Medicine, 13*(5), 617–621.

Yassin, A., Mostafa, M. A., & Moawad, M. K. (1966). Cerumen and its microchemical analysis. *Journal of Laryngology and Otology, 80,* 933–938.

Yoshiura, K., Kinoshita, A., Ishida, T., Ninokata, A., Ishikawa, T., Kaname, T., . . . Niikawa, N. (2006). A SNP in the ABCC11 gene is the determinant of human earwax type. *Natural Genetics, 38*(3), 324–330.

Zackaria, M., & Aymat, A. (2009). Ear candling: A case report. *European Journal of General Practice, 15*(3), 168–169.

Zemplenyi, J., Gilman, S., & Dirks, D. (1985). Optical method for measurement of ear canal length. *Journal of the Acoustical Society of America, 78*(4), 2146–2148.

Zikk, D., Rapoport, Y., & Himelfarb, M. Z. (1991). Invasive external otitis after removal of impacted cerumen by irrigation [Letter]. *New England Journal of Medicine, 325,* 969–970.

Zivic, R. C., & King, S. (1993). Cerumen-impaction management for clients of all ages. *Nurse Practitioner, 18,* 29, 33–36, 39.

Zwislocki, J. J. (1957). Some measurements of the impedance at the eardrum. *Journal of the Acoustical Society of America, 29,* 349–356.

Zwislocki, J. J. (1970). *An acoustic coupler for earphone calibration.* Special report LSC-S-7, Laboratory of Sensory Communication, Syracuse University.

Zwislocki, J. J. (1971). *An acoustic coupler for earphone calibration.* Special report LSC-S-9, Laboratory of Sensory Communication, Syracuse University.

Zwislocki, J. J. (1980). An ear simulatory for acoustic measurements: Rationale, principles, and limitations. In G. A. Studebacker & I. Hochberg (Eds.), *Acoustical factors affecting hearing aid performance* (pp. 127–147). Baltimore, MD: University Park Press.

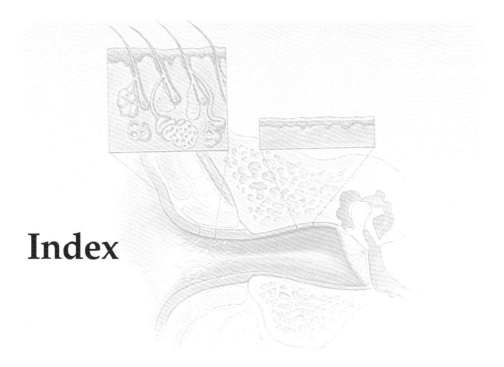

Index